UNBORN JESUS OUR HOPE

by

George A. Peate

Foreword by Ronda Chervin, Ph.D.

Life Cycle Books
Niagara Falls, NY • Toronto, ON

Scripture quotes used in this book are from the Revised Standard Version Catholic Edition. Some quotes, from the King James Version, are distinguished by KJV. Some quotes, from the New American Bible, are distinguished by NAB.

Published by:

Life Cycle Books
PO Box 1008
Niagara Falls, NY 14304-1008

Phone: (800) 214-5849
Fax: (888) 690-8532
e-mail: orders@lifecyclebooks.com
www.lifecyclebooks.com

Canadian office:
Life Cycle Books Ltd.
421 Nugget Ave. Unit 8
Toronto, ON M1S 4L8

Printed in Canada

ISBN # 0-919225-31-4

CONTENTS

Acknowledgements		v
Foreword		vii
Introduction		xi
Prologue		xv
Chapter One	The Incarnation: One Cell and One With Us	1
Chapter Two	Journey To the Hill Country of Judea	17
Chapter Three	Exchange Of Prophetic Greetings	37
Chapter Four	The Visitation: A Three Month Retreat	55
Chapter Five	The Return To Nazareth	75
Chapter Six	Joseph Accepts Jesus as His Own Son	87
Chapter Seven	The First Christian Family	103
Chapter Eight	Sent By God to Bethlehem	121
Chapter Nine	The Great Nativity	137
Epilogue	On Praying to Unborn Jesus	153
Appendix I	Identity and Personhood of the Incarnate Son of God	159
Appendix II	Prayers Honoring the Incarnation of Jesus Christ	163
Appendix III	The "Hail Mary" Prayer	169

I dedicate this book to all those who have lovingly helped unborn children and their mothers (directly through services or indirectly through education and other important efforts), to all those unborn babies known to you the reader now during the time while you read this book and to all unborn babies at risk. . .

Acknowledgements

I am deeply indebted to Bridget Neumayr and Ronda Chervin who reviewed early drafts of this book and offered valuable assistance. Bridget's editorial advice and Ronda's literary suggestions were instrumental to bringing the project to completion.

The book took more than one and a half decades to write and I have probably come to appreciate more than most the blessing of encouragement given by others. I offer a heartfelt thanks to ALL my family members, friends and spiritual benefactors who offered encouragement and prayer as I meandered along on this journey. Since the most recent years were the more difficult ones, my gratitude is all the more fresh in my mind and heart. Thanks to: Judie Brown, Licia Nicassio, Geri Urrutia, Gina and Mike Farrell, Professor Donald DeMarco, Fr. Paul A. Donlan, Fr. James M. Kubicki, S.J., Fernando H. Uribe, Most Reverend Bishop Robert F. Vasa and those others who are victims of my poor memory.

A special thanks to my publisher Paul Broughton (a pioneer in providing pro-life materials to the world's Respect Life movement) and my diligent editors Erin and Scott Nicholson.

A most loving thank you to my mother Mary Peate for her enthusiasm, to my children and daughter-in-law for their understanding and other related virtues, and finally to my wife Michele for her patience and support over the years and whose dedication and hard work on this project in these most recent years has been inspirational to me.

May God bless you all and always.

FOREWORD

"Surely Unborn Jesus had – and has – a special place in His most tiny hidden heart for today's vulnerable unborn children." Epilogue, *Unborn Jesus Our Hope*.

What are the chances of reading a pro-life book with a hopeful and even exalted message? That was my initial skeptical approach when my friend, George Peate, agreed to let me look at a manuscript he was preparing called *Unborn Jesus Our Hope*. But first, let me back up to share some key memories of my own pro-life journey that help explain my reaction to Peate's book.

I was born in 1937 to parents who loved and cared for me and my twin-sister, but whose philosophy of life did not allow for any unconditional affirmation of the intrinsic worth of the human person. Part of my conversion at the age of 21 to Catholic Christianity was the recognition that a baby in the womb was more valuable than a book on a shelf. Years later, while I was a professor of philosophy at Loyola Marymount University of Los Angeles, I became part of the pro-life movement both in the teaching of ethics and by praying in front of abortuaries. And my husband, Martin Chervin, wrote a play Born/Unborn depicting the grief of a father becoming aware that the mother of their child is going for a late-term abortion.

It was in front of an abortuary, in 1982, that I first met my fellow pro-life friends George and Michele Peate and their family. There was much sharing of wisdom amongst the quietly praying protesters between counseling women coming for abortions. I remember once someone said that the mystery of Mary's visitation to Elizabeth showed how the babe in the womb was a person. There in Scripture we didn't read about how two not yet human salamander-like swimmers waved their tails in greeting but about how the unborn tiny person of Jesus blessed the tiny unborn person John.

Another memory – I was sitting at the edge of my seat in a movie theatre thrilling to the image of that small man, Gandhi, defying the British Empire with prayer and non-violent resistance. I asked loudly as that great film ended, "Don't the lives of the babies in the womb mean as much to us as the welfare of his people meant to Gandhi? Where are leaders in our movement who love God and unborn babies with that degree of sacrificial fervor?" Within a month I heard of the early attempts of Operation Rescue led by such heroic deeply Christian believers as Joan Andrews.

When I finally got to read a draft of *Unborn Jesus Our Hope*, I thought that only a parent could write so lovingly about the process of life in the womb, mingling this awe with a presentation of theological truth, so scholarly and yet vibrant. I was stunned with joy at the beauty of Peate's account of the meaning for us of unborn Jesus.

I see now that part of my interest in the manuscript had to do with burn-out. After years of activism in the pro-life movement I had become tired of reading protest articles. I needed to spend any time left over from teaching, writing and speaking in quiet prayer. I did not know how to bring the anger, hurt and disappointment about abortion into that inner sanctuary of the heart of Jesus or into soothing recitation of the mysteries of His life given in the rosary.

But now, reading *Unborn Jesus Our Hope* in its final form I am deeply moved. I see how just as the errors of radical feminism challenged us to develop a true Christian sense of womanhood, so can the scourge of abortion bring forth new wonder about the unborn person in the light of the life of the unborn Jesus.

Unborn Jesus Our Hope is a masterpiece. With its poetic style and theologically sound presentation, it provides a unique synthesis of contemplation and human experience. Studded with evocative quotations, the reader is invited to commune with the great perceptions of centuries of Church teachers. While written from a Catholic background, I believe all Christians will love this book, especially because of the constant references to Scripture.

Simple reflections gently challenge us as we read. Peate writes about the visitation of Mary to her cousin Elizabeth, that "Mary acts with God at His prompt and pace." At His prompt and pace. . . I ask myself, do I act with God at his prompt and pace or do I rush ahead and then beg God to grace my impetuous sometimes misguided deeds?

Thank you, Holy Spirit, for Your light shining in the darkness of the culture of death, upon the mind of George Peate, who has written this refreshingly beautiful reflection: *Unborn Jesus Our Hope.*

Ronda Chervin, Ph.D., is a professor of philosophy, a widow and grandmother, and author of numerous books about Christian living.

Introduction

Welcome to the Church's first devotion – devotion to Unborn Jesus! God invites us into this intimate and personal devotion of Mary, directed towards her unborn Son and Savior Jesus Christ, because He wants us to discover anew many wonderful things about our Lord's Incarnation and our own personal redemption. But in a special way in this modern time, God the Father wants to show humanity how much He loves unborn children. The Father sends His unborn Son to deliver an important message to a people who have lost their way.

Unborn Jesus is the way! In the hiddenness of His mother's womb Unborn Jesus is already on His mission to save fallen humanity. This is the unspoken gospel before the Gospel preached by our Savior during His public ministry – a hidden unnoticed gospel, but a gospel nonetheless. Do not disdain this unspoken gospel as many disdain the unspoken stories of unborn children today. The kingdom of God is like a buried treasure (Mt 13:44). Here in the womb, for nine months, Jesus is this buried treasure. Here is the embryonic kingdom of God before the manifested Kingdom of God – a tiny realm, but holy and full of abundant graces for Christians of good will.

For nine months of longing Jesus is unborn, undiscovered, unknown and even unwanted – loving us first, reaching out to us even before birth, whispering from His tiny uncharted heart an unspoken word: Love! The first word of the ballad of our salvation. Yet, today our civilization is embracing a "culture of death", intent on discrediting unborn children, stripping them of their humanity and personhood and taking their lives for the sake of expediency. Many of us are terribly discouraged by this, but we must remind ourselves of St. Paul's teaching: "...but where sin increased, grace abounded all the more..." (Rom 5:20).

Where is grace abounding in our present world for unborn children? The answer is: Unborn Jesus. In his book *The Son of Man*, Francois Mauriac said that he places himself "on the side of childhood" and "above all, on the side of the infant God", and he also spoke of God not only as Eternal Father, but also as "Eternal Child". Isn't this what our modern world needs? Let us put ourselves squarely on the side of Christ the Child, returning to the beginning of Christ's Incarnation, to the foundation of Christianity, to explore and discover that initial stage of the childhood mission of God on earth – Christ the Lord in the womb of His mother.

The pregnancy of Mary – no longer "too holy" to talk about, is now too relevant to ignore. This book is a spiritual presentation of the life of the greatest unborn child that ever lived. Our study will not dwell on the sin and negativity of abortion, but on the grace which abounds in the secret life of Unborn Jesus. Not exactly a spiritual ultrasound of His first nine months, but a reflection on the life, identity, glory and mission of Unborn Jesus.

I have tried to focus exclusively on Unborn Jesus, but I am sure the reader will forgive me for stumbling across the maternal love of His mother, and commenting on that providential unity of their lives and purposes as well. Given the subject matter of this book, I found it somewhat difficult to separate the One from the other. The unborn baby Jesus embodies a divine sparked love from heaven which is complemented by a maternal love sparked from earth. Speaking for humanity, poet William Wordsworth described Mary as our "solitary boast" partly because she welcomed our Lord into the world on our behalf with a humble, open and overflowing heart. ("The Virgin", Ecclesiastical Sonnet XXV…).

Many ancient prophecies were fulfilled within the womb, the body and the family of Mary, and their fulfillments were holy in every respect. Perhaps we can discover anew the awesome meaning and power of these prophecies from the new and fresh perspective of Unborn Jesus. As we witness in faith their fulfillment by Jesus (and His mother), we can know Him better, while also growing in our appreciation of every unborn child – created in the likeness and image of the Almighty – who is created to fulfill the promise and plan of God.

Many unborn children today have few friends. Enter Unborn Jesus, the best friend of each unborn child. Now that the unborn are fiercely persecuted and disdained, the first unborn child comes to be identified with them completely, in every possible way. And He calls out to the Church to be discovered, understood and loved. Does God love unborn children? Unborn Jesus answered that question for nine months and forever.

Throughout human history there has only been one redemptive pregnancy. Eve's first pregnancy, with Cain, was a prototypical pregnancy, but was not a redemptive pregnancy. When Abraham's wife Sarah was pregnant with Isaac it was a pregnancy of promise and destiny, but not redemptive. When famous mothers or mothers of famous children were pregnant their pregnancies were perhaps remarkable or noteworthy, but not redemptive. And when your mother was pregnant with you, it was a very special pregnancy, but not redemptive. Only the pregnancy of Mary of Nazareth was, in every sense of the word, Redemptive: a pregnancy which Christians can discover by faith, and in our present age must discover.

Right from the start, and providentially so, the Incarnation and the redemptive pregnancy of Mary the mother of Unborn Jesus are filled with hope from on high. A hushed whisper of hope for undeserving humanity. Hope for every family. Hope for every mother. Hope for every unborn child. In a world gone mad and running away from God, let us now turn with expectation to Unborn Jesus our hope.

Prologue

You are my son, today I have begotten you.
Psalm 2:7 and Hebrews 1:5

The Son of God is eternal. As the ancient Christian Nicene Creed (formulated in 325 A.D.) says, "eternally begotten of the Father". The Navarre Bible Commentary explains the word "today" as used in the above psalm as begotten "in the continuous present of the eternal Godhead".[1] So Christ is eternally begotten of the Father before He is temporally born of Mary.

If we want to probe this mystery a bit further, we might recall that Christ is begotten within or from the Father's "bosom" or "heart". John the Evangelist proclaims "the only begotten Son, which is in the bosom of the Father" (Jn 1:18, KJV). The term "bosom" is now antiquated so some biblical translations, such as the New English Bible (NEB), translate the original Greek term κολπον as the "Father's heart".

We might say that Christ is begotten from the "womb-like" heart of God the Father eternally and then temporally born from the "heart-like" womb of His mother. Just as the physical womb is meant to expand with life, St. Josemaria Escriva points out that the spiritual heart is meant to expand with love.[2] *At* any rate, both the plan of salvation and the idea of Unborn Jesus also originate, in a sense, within the eternal heart of Almighty God.

We now step down from the eternal perspective to human history proper – skipping like skimming stones across history's wave tops – from Eden, to the Mediterranean region, to the promised land, to Nazareth. History unfolding in every direction, every which way, a multiplicity of races, religions, philosophies, governments, with waves of civilizations swelling up, then collapsing, to be replaced by new ones. Three civilizations are of particular note: Hebrew, Roman and Greek.

Through a providential confluence of these civilizations, God created the ideal circumstances for the Messiah's coming. While Greeks and Romans were developing communications and transportation networks throughout the civilized world, Jews were dispersing throughout the empire and establishing viable synagogue communities. A morally exhausted pagan world was prepared to receive the invigorating and creative message of the one true God. The time was ripe. God worked "... according to his purpose which he set forth in Christ as a plan for the fullness of time..." (Eph 1:9-10).

Within Israel two prophetic promises were being realized. First, the Messiah was anticipated. The Jews knew he would be from the tribe of Judah and later understood he would also be from the house of David. Secondly, as promised by the prophets, God was secretly forming faithful believers in a remnant community: the priest Zechariah and his wife Elizabeth and their unborn son John (Lk 1.5-25, 39-80), Simeon (Lk 2.25-35), Anna (Lk 2.36-38), of course Joseph (Mt 1) and most importantly Mary. One writer, Maria Boulding, has spoken of Israel at that time in history as an expectant "womb-community" awaiting the Messiah.[3]

Joseph, a town carpenter of Nazareth, was engaged to a young woman in the town named Mary. We all know the story more or less. Together they had come to a defining point in their lives – a personal "fullness of time" shared by both of them. They were ready for each other and ready for God. And soon God would be ready for them, but not yet.

To best appreciate the final months and days leading up to the Incarnation, let us focus on Mary and reflect on some possible aspects of her faith life, particularly with reference to the great commandment: "Hear, O Israel: The Lord our God is one Lord; and you shall love the Lord your God with all your heart, and with all your soul, and with all your might" (Deut 6:4-5).

This command instructs one to give one's entirety, in love offering all to God. The word "all" is employed three times. The last line "with all your might" (the Hebrew word translated as "might" has also been translated as "strength") is meant to suggest a comprehensive list of the vital characteristics of one's mental and physical make-up: all one's spiritual and corporal abilities. (See Jesus' reference to this command; Mk 12:29-30.)

Someone as spiritually astute as Mary would likely begin each day with an offering of herself in the spirit of the foregoing great command – a morning offering of her entire self, if you will perhaps with an attitude somewhat akin to that expressed years later by the apostle Paul: "…present your bodies as a living sacrifice, holy and acceptable to God, which is your spiritual worship" (Rom 12:1).

We are confident that Mary's habitual offering of herself to God must have been "holy and acceptable" because the Archangel Gabriel stated that she had "found favor with God". Mary's gift to God was all encompassing and absolute, an utter dispossessing of all she was and all that she had to give: a pure heart, singleness of mind, faithfulness, youthful desire and energy, feminine nature, fertility and virginity and all her other personal and spiritual attributes. God accepted her goodwill offering of herself while respecting her free will and biological nature.

Providence waited for a particular ovulation of Mary's body. God chose Mary from "before the foundation of the world" (Eph 1:4), God had specially consecrated and prepared Mary in singular fashion from the very foundation of her own life – that is from the first cell of her existence.[4] God had waited for entire civilizations and empires to shift and change with time: now God could also wait for a biological fertility cycle to catch up with His designs. Though Mary's ovaries released but one ovum each month, her heart was more fertile by a hundredfold, presenting numerous holy intentions and desires to the Lord daily. And so she prepared herself for the unknown will of God. She represented the "first fruits" of her generation and her people as she waited upon God Most High.

On that immortal day in human history when, unbeknownst to any earthly creature, the body of Mary was presenting its own offering – releasing an ovum into the fallopian tube – Mary remained steadfast and open to God. Like the "first fruits" of a harvest the Israelites were required to offer in sacrifice, this ovum – the fruit of Mary's body – was ripe, unblemished and pleasing to God. The ovum traveled slowly down the fallopian tube towards Mary's womb. It was now "the fullness of time"….

PROLOGUE ENDNOTES

1. Jose Maria Casciaro et al., ed., *The Navarre Bible; The Epistle of Hebrews,* trans.James Gavigan et al. (Dublin, Ireland: Four Courts Press, 1991), 57.
2. St. Josemaria Escriva, *The Way of the Cross* (New York: Scepter, 1990), 76.
3. Maria Boulding, *The Coming of God* (London: SPCK, 1982), 3.
4. *The Catechism of the Catholic Church* #484-511, provides an overview of traditional teaching regarding the Immaculate Conception of Mary and her privileged relationship to Jesus Christ. For example, #492: "The 'splendor of an entirely unique holiness' by which Mary is 'enriched from the first instant of her conception' comes wholly from Christ: she is 'redeemed, in a more exalted fashion, by reason of the merits of her son.' The Father blessed Mary more than any other created person 'in Christ with every spiritual blessing in the heavenly places' and chose her 'in Christ before the foundation of the world, to be holy and blameless before him in love'." Circa 415 A.D. St. Augustine referred to Mary's unique position in his work *Corrections (Nature and Grace).* For a more in depth discussion of Mary's privileged position and role see *The Mother of the Saviour and Our Interior Life* by Fr. Reginald Garrigou-Lagrange, O.P. (Published by Tan Books, 1993).

1

The Incarnation: One Cell And One With Us

Lift up your heads, O gates!
and be lifted up, O ancient doors!
that the King of glory may come in.
Who is this King of glory?
The Lord of hosts, he is the King of glory!
Psalm 24:9-10

The Lord had promised repeatedly that He would come to deliver His people. But how would it happen? The above psalm calls to mind a triumphant king riding victoriously into a city fortress, a scene of banners waving, horses bearing gallant soldiers, shining swords raised high, shields glistening in the noon day sun, trumpets, horns, shouts of joy, even dancing in the streets!

But God in His infinite wisdom chose a more marvelous way for His entrance among the children of Adam and Eve: "In the sixth month the angel Gabriel was sent from God to a city of Galilee named Nazareth, to a virgin betrothed to a man whose name was Joseph, of the house of David; and the virgin's name was Mary" (Lk 1:26-27).

Nazareth was a small town of no consequence, mentioned neither "in the Old Testament writings nor in those of the historian Josephus".[1] Joseph, a carpenter, while respected for his craftsmanship, fairness in business dealings and pleasant nature, was merely a poor tradesman trying to scratch out a living. His royal lineage was largely forgotten, covered now in sawdust, obscured in humbled generations of sinners and peasants since the glory days of King David. The young woman was likely more obscure than the town carpenter. Gabriel was sent to a nobody, who had next to nothing, and who lived in the middle of nowhere. Or so it would seem. "And he came to her and said, 'Hail, full of grace, the Lord is with you!'" (Lk 1:28).

Why would an angel show such reverence towards a human being? Why would Gabriel standing "in the presence of God" (Lk 1:19), speak in this way? He himself answers the question: because she had "found favor with God" (Lk 1:30). What was this "favor" which was found in Mary? As Father Faber wrote:

> What was it in her which so attracted God? What drew the Word from the Bosom of the Father into her Bosom with such mysterious allurement? It was as if he were following the shadow of his own beauty. It was because the delights of the Holy Trinity were so faithfully imaged there. All was his. It was to his own he went. It was his own which drew him. . .Her natural life was his own idea, her beauty a sparkle of his science. . .Her graces were all from him. She had nothing which she had not received. Like the moon, her loveliness was all from borrowed light. . .[2]

When Gabriel appeared to Mary perhaps she was at prayer in her home, or as Faber says, "in an hour of awestricken worship".[3] The dialogue between Gabriel and Mary is fascinating, but since this scene has been the subject of countless sermons and thousands of books over the past two thousand years, we will not study it extensively here. Suffice it to say that Mary received her angelic visitor and his message with simple humility, energetic obedience, and a consuming desire to serve God. Harriet Beecher Stowe points to another noteworthy quality found in Mary:

> There is in her whole character a singular poise and calmness. When the Angel of the Annunciation appeared to her she was not overcome by the presence of the spiritual being as Daniel was, who records that "he fell on his face and there was no strength in him." Mary, in calm and firm simplicity, looks the angel in the face, and ponders what the wonderful announcement may mean. When she finds that it really does mean that she, a poor lonely maiden, is the chosen woman of all the human race – the gainer of the crown of which every Jewish woman had dreamed for ages – she is still calm.[4]

The Manner and Moment of the Incarnation

> *"The Holy Spirit will come upon you, and the power of the Most High will overshadow you..."*
>
> Luke 1:34

It has generally been held that this overshadowing by the Holy Spirit occurred immediately after Mary gave her verbal acceptance to the angelic proposal: "Behold, I am the handmaid of the Lord; let it be to me according to your word" (Lk 1:38), either while the angel Gabriel was still there or immediately after his departure. Of the miraculous conception of Jesus Christ, St. Thomas Aquinas (1225-1274) observes: "It behooved His body to develop in the same way as the bodies of other men, so as to prove the reality of His human nature. For if we consider in this conception anything connected with the matter thereof, which was supplied by the mother, it was in all such things natural..."[5]

Typically, fertilization occurs in one of the two fallopian tubes as the woman's ovum travels through that tube toward the uterus. We can probably assume that the conception of our Lord occurred in this same manner and location.[6]

The prodigious Father Faber describes "the power of the Most High" overshadowing Mary: "The jubilant ocean of Uncreated Love rose like a cloud, and hung with His deluge of graces and gifts over the kneeling maiden..."[7] "...and the divine complacency rolled above her in majestic peals of soft, mysterious thunder, and a God-like Shadow falls upon her for a moment...Her head sank upon her bosom, and her soul lay down in a silence which was like the peace of God. The Word was made flesh."[8]

Here Faber attempts to express the inexpressible: the intimate supernatural moment of the Incarnation of the Son of God. St. Bonaventure (1221-1274) provides us with yet another perspective on this singular and marvelous event:

> For you must know that the sublime work of the Incarnation was the work of the whole Trinity, although it was only the Person of the Son of God who became incarnate. It was as if one who put on a tunic were helped by two standing on either side of him who held the tunic in their hands....For although the Holy Trinity is everywhere, nevertheless you must think of It in your meditation as being

> here in a very special manner, by reason of the great and unique work which is being done.[9]

Unimaginable beforehand, incomprehensible afterward: the Incarnation is a glorious crowning to all of human history. In a reversal of the creation of Eve from Adam's side, here Mary could say on behalf of all humanity: "The Son of God is bone of our bone, and flesh of our flesh!"[10] By divine intervention this is the beginning of the new creation in Christ (II Cor.5:17, Rev.21:5) as Frank Sheed writes:

> In the sense that other human beings have a mother and father, He had a mother only. The bodies of other human beings result from the action of an element supplied by their father upon an element supplied by their mother. In the case of our Lord the effect upon the female element normally produced by the male element was produced simply by a creative act of the will of God. Thus He is a member of Adam's race on His mother's side; He is a Jew on His mother's side; but not upon His father's side, for in the order of human generation He had no father.[11]

By divine intervention, God created for Himself a human body and from the first moment of His physical existence, in modern terms the one cell stage, the world's greatest mystery is truly man. That first cell – the great first cell of the new creation – is the cornerstone of the temple of our Lord's Body! It was the cornerstone that the "builders" would reject (Mt 21:42), but which Mary accepted with all of her heart. Evangelist and Pastor Jack Hayford puts it in perspective: "I think there can be no question: The most surprised person in human history was a maiden named Mary....The Mary miracle is the fountainhead miracle; it's the beginning of all God's wonder-works of redemption....It didn't start in a manger in Bethlehem, but in a womb in Nazareth."[12]

Exactly what occurred at the miracle moment of the Incarnation is something we need to consider thoughtfully. One seventeenth century mystic who wrote extensively about the Incarnation, Mary of Agreda, explains that:

> ....in one instant, four things happened. First, the most holy body of Christ our Lord was formed...Secondly, the most holy soul of the same Lord was created, just as the other souls. Thirdly, the soul and the body united in order to compose his perfect humanity. Fourthly,

> the Divinity united Itself in the Person of the Word with the humanity, which together became one composite being in hypostatical union; and thus was formed Christ true God and Man, our Lord and Redeemer. . . .all that substantially belonged to this divine mystery. . . .happened and was completed in one act or instant; so that we cannot say that in any moment of time Christ our highest Good was only man. For from the first instant He was man and true God; as soon as his humanity arrived at being man, He was also God; therefore He could not at any time be called a mere man, nor for one instant; but from the very beginning He was God-man. . . .[13]

It can truly be said that the glory of our Lord's Incarnation is so far above us, that saints, theologians, evangelists and mystics alike can only grapple with it one aspect at a time. But let us remember that the context for our reflection on this great mystery is always that of a personal act of divine love.

One Cell and One with Us

But Who is this that comes into ordinary human history by such extraordinary means? What manner of person is this? How are we to understand Him and relate to Him? C. S. Lewis explains:

> The Eternal Being, who knows everything and who created the whole universe, became not only a man but (before that) a baby, and before that a foetus inside a Woman's body. If you want to get the hang of it, think how you would like to become a slug or a crab. The result of this was that you now had one man who really was what all men were intended to be: one man in whom the created life, derived from his Mother, allowed itself to be completely and perfectly turned into the begotten life. The natural human creature in Him was taken up fully into the divine Son. Thus in one instance humanity had, so to speak, arrived: had passed into the life of Christ.[14]

And so the Christian era begins with the historical Jesus, and the historical Jesus begins here and now in the Incarnation as humanity "passed into the life of Christ." And in a special way the sanctification of the unborn human state begins immediately. By taking on this unborn human identity, this miniscule cross of human passage, He hallows it, and will do so every day for nine months. His time in the womb will not be wasted. Just as a martyr's blood leaves a prophetic and inspirational trail of fidelity to the will of God, so too this time of divine humiliation enhances the dignity of all future unborn babies. After Unborn Jesus, all unborn babies have a greater claim to be born, and then born again. "Since therefore the children share in flesh and blood, he himself likewise partook of the same nature. . . .he had to be made like his brethren in every respect. . ." (Heb 2:14, 17).

Because He completely identifies with all unborn children, indeed is one of them, when we lift up and exalt Unborn Jesus, in a real sense we lift up all unborn children with Him. Him we honor as God, they we honor as children created in His image and for His glory. As we contemplate Him in the womb for the next nine months, we shall learn that in fact Unborn Jesus is the champion of all unborn children. And when we praise Unborn Jesus we strike a spiritual blow at the very core of a perverse culture of death.

Note: The reader is encouraged to read Appendix I to supplement this discussion of the Incarnation. Appendix I devotes just over two pages to examining the identity and personhood of the Incarnate Son of God from a theological viewpoint. Reflecting upon the mystery of Jesus Christ in more theologically precise terms helps us to better understand His mission and actions within the womb. It is to one of these profound acts – indeed His very first act – to which we now turn.

Our Lord's First Act In Utero

Our Lord's first words – uttered from the womb – are not recorded in any of the Gospels, but in the book of Hebrews. The first act of Jesus Christ after His Incarnation is a prayer offering Himself and His human body to the Father:

> *Consequently, when Christ came into the world, he said,*
> *"Sacrifices and offerings thou hast not desired,*
> *but a body hast thou prepared for me;*
> *in burnt offerings and sin offerings*
> *thou hast taken no pleasure.*
> *Then I said, "Lo, I have come to do Thy will, O God,'*
> *as it is written of me in the roll of the book." (Heb 10:5-7)*

These words (foretold in Psalm 40) – are the only words known to be spoken by Unborn Jesus (or by any unborn child for that matter).[15] Pope Paul VI referred to this prayer as "the fundamental offering that the Incarnate Word made to the Father when He entered the world"[16] The point here is that this prayer was not offered prior to the Incarnation but rather after it had occurred.

Many spiritual writers and theologians hold that this prayer was offered immediately upon Christ's entry into the world. This prayer would seem to be associated with that first moment of the Incarnation; probably at the one cell stage. St. Ignatius of Loyola (1491-1556) tells us: "A Man-God who, from the first moment of His conception, offers Himself to His Father. This is to teach us that there is not a single moment of our lives that does not belong to God."[17]

And The International Bible Commentary explains: "Here, then, the words of the psalmist become the words of the incarnate Son, overheard as they were spoken to the Father".[18] It is with such childlike faith and understanding that we can best grasp the significance of this original prayer communication of Unborn Jesus.

Priest and Victim Both

How appropriate that our Lord's first words were a prayer to His Father. Consider the words of Blessed Columba Marmion:

> "We ought not to consider Christ's Sacrifice as offered only at the time of the Passion. Christ is a Victim from the moment of the Incarnation, and it is as Victim that He offers Himself.... He accepted to fulfill all that was decreed: He said to His Father: "Behold I come": *Ecce venio.* The initial act of offering whereby He wholly yielded Himself up, virtually contained all His sacrifice...."[19]

Let us not view the words of this prayer and their implied meaning in a morbid light. Rather let us understand that this prayer – and indeed the Incarnation itself – is born of a great enduring love for all of creation, and especially for fallen humanity. The sobering commentary above helps us see clearly the straight road Jesus traveled from conception through crucifixion to resurrection. It gives a new and deeper meaning to Isaiah's quote about the Suffering Servant; "...I have set my face like a flint..." (Is 50:7) Yes, even from the womb.

"But a body hast thou prepared for me. . ."

Our first impression might incline us to think that Christ at the one cell stage of human development doesn't yet have a body "prepared" for Him, that it will be prepared in the future. However, this is not the case. At this one cell stage He has a tiny body that contains within it the whole physiological make up and mystery of His humanity that will flourish and grow with time. At this one cell stage, the King of Glory Who is robed in majesty takes on the simple garment of a creature – human flesh – and is now clothed with humility. His humanity is His humility.

From the one cell stage to His reddened, bruised and scourged frame struggling under the wooden cross, and then upon it, this is the One Body to be offered lovingly for our sins. All the sin offerings of past centuries had come to naught. But now there is finally something worth offering. Though the time according to God's plan has not yet arrived.

Infinitely small now, but in half a lifespan, infinitely ripe. Let this Body develop into full manhood, let this Son of Man lead a perfect and sinless life, let Him redefine love and unleash a Spirit of forgiveness and healing, let His lips reveal the innermost truths about human life and then, see Him "...present (His Body) as a living sacrifice, holy and acceptable to God, which is (His) spiritual worship" (Rom 12:1).

But before Golgotha, He begins His offering to God the Father here in His mother's womb. Mary's womb has now become "the place" in the scheme of things: the focal point of creation and the place where Christ initially does God's will. The reformer, John Calvin, sees the womb of Mary for what it is: "Choosing from the womb of the Virgin a temple for his residence, He who was the Son of God, became also the Son of Man."[20]

Mary's womb has become a holy temple. In a temple we meet God. It is a place to worship God. We also go there to pray, to converse with God and to listen to God. Indeed and as it is sometimes put: "to be alone with God". In the temple of Mary's womb, we witness both the sacred presence of God as well as the sacred acts being performed there by Unborn Jesus.

Before the time of Christ the Israelites built a tabernacle in which the Ark of the Covenant was sheltered. Later the Ark of the Covenant was kept in the holy Temple in Jerusalem, until the destruction of that Temple in 587 B.C. The Ark of the Covenant seems to have been lost during the following period of the Babylonian Exile. But now with the Incarnation, here is the new Ark of the New Covenant and the womb of Mary is transformed according to the Divine Will and purposes. Cardinal Berulle (1575-1629), founder of the French School of Spirituality sums up this concept well: "He is in her as in a temple where He praises and adores God; where He offers His respects to the eternal Father, not only for Himself but for every creature. It is a holy and sacred temple where Jesus dwells, the true ark of the true covenant. It is the first and holiest temple of Jesus."[21]

The incarnate life of Jesus Christ begins a liturgy: The liturgy of the life of our Lord. And it is a living liturgy. Christ as victim brings forward His Body – one unique, living human cell, literally the first fruits of His Incarnation – so that the first act of the redemption plan begins at the first moment of His Incarnation. Immediately Christ as Priest offers the one and only acceptable sacrifice to the Most High God. Indeed, words fall short, but this liturgy of oblation inaugurating our salvation is a most profound aspect of the Incarnation.

"Lo, I have come to do Thy will, O God. . ."

These words of Our Lord – this prayer offering of Himself – reveal to us the unwavering purpose of His entire life, a mission statement explaining why He has come into the world and what lies ahead of Him. It is a battle cry from the first instant of His life, and one all Christians would do well to heed.

As we know by our own experience, "the spirit is willing but the flesh is weak." But as our Lord came into our world, He embodied the fullest harmony between spirit and flesh, between God's will and the body. His was a wholeness and integrity unknown, unfathomable, and as yet unborn. And from the outset He was clothed in the incarnational virtues of humility and obedience. The first humans had bodies created from earth. They had a type of "original humility" prior to their temptation by the devil and subsequent fall. The root word "humus" – meaning earth – points out the meaning of the word humility. We now witness a Divine humility on the part of the second person of the Blessed Trinity in this initial moment of His Incarnation, as He comes down to earth.

From His coming into the world, He offers this wholesome unity of His body and His soul, and the full concord of his human will with his Divine Will, so that in Him the restoration of the human race begins. He is already the "new" eldest brother of a renewing humanity, and, as such, has even now begun the overthrow of the legacy of that former "eldest brother", Cain. He is the obedient Son. Theologian Hans Urs von Balthasar wrote: "At the beginning of all his work there is found obedience: the readiness to let himself be disposed of by the Father according to his total will. . . .Already the way from the bosom of the eternal Father to the womb of the temporal Mother is a path of obedience, the most difficult and consequential of ways, but one which is trod on mission from the Father."[22]

Perhaps St. Paul best captures the essence of our Lord's humility and obedience in the famous passage from his letter to the Philippians (2:5-8): ". . .though he was in the form of God, did not count equality with God a thing to be grasped, but emptied himself, taking the form of a servant, being born in the likeness of men. And being found in human form he humbled himself and became obedient unto death, even death on a cross."

This teaching has not been lost on Christians through the centuries. Paul helps us to better understand the words of Unborn Jesus in Hebrews 10 and the nature of the offering and commitment being thereby expressed. In those words of Unborn Jesus we find the kernel of 1. a theology of the body, 2. a spirituality of the body, and 3. an attitude of respect for life and the human body. Unborn Jesus views the body prepared for Him as a gift from the Father which expresses the relationship between Him and His Father. One's body and life are prepared for a purpose. The will of the Creator is the key to one's existence, both in the general broad sense of one's life, as well as in the everyday minutiae of daily experience.

Earlier, reference was made to Jesus referring to himself as that cornerstone which would be rejected by the builders. Recall that the first cell of our Lord's unborn Body was the cornerstone of the Temple of our Lord's Body. Both Isaiah (Is 28:16) and Peter (I Pet 2:4-6) describe that cornerstone as "chosen and precious". At the one cell stage of existence His Body is "chosen" for God's will, though Mary is the only creature who knew it as "precious" at this initial point. In the months ahead, from this one cell the completely formed body of Jesus will be prepared. A tiny heart with which to love others, a brain to fathom truth's meaning, small hands to reach out and embrace both friend and stranger, little feet to begin the sojourn of life, eyes to take in creation and a mouth to speak the Gospel.

Sacred Words of Consecration

The Incarnation and the crucifixion are two expressions of the same love, the same humility, the same disposition to do the will of the Father. Indeed words of consecration accompany both acts of the Son of God.

At the beginning of His earthly life, as Our Lord takes a human body for Himself in His Incarnation, He says to His Father:

> "...but a body hast Thou prepared for me...'Lo, I have come to do Thy will, O God'" (Heb 10:5,7)

Many years later as He prepares for the end of His earthly life, and takes leave of His disciples, He says:

> "This is my body which is given for you." (Lk 22:19)

Monsignor Robert Hugh Benson has developed this theme:

> Thus, in that last emphatic act of the life of His Humiliation He took Bread, and cried, not Here is my Essential Self, but 'This is my Body which is given for you,' since that Body was the instrument of Redemption. And, if the Christian claim is to be believed, this act was but a continuation (though in another sense) of that first act known as the Incarnation. He who leaned over the Bread at that "last sad Supper with His own" had, in another but similar manner, leaned over Mary herself with similar words upon His lips.[23]

At the last supper Jesus speaks of His approaching fulfillment of the Father's will by which He will take that same body set aside and prepared for Him at conception, to a place prepared for the ultimate offering of His redemptive body at Golgotha. (But first He will establish a way for all those members of His mystical Body to thereafter physically/mystically receive – and even eat – His Body, Jn.6:51-58.) Very conscious of this act of submission to the Father's will, He walks to the Garden of Gethsemane, a garden like Eden where His human ancestors had abandoned the holy will of God, and there offers Himself, His Life, His Body to the Father. In a sweat of blood the perfect harmony between His will and body and between His human will and divine will seems to falter. He prays three times the ultimate prayer, perhaps in reparation for the threefold definitive sins of Eve, Adam, and Cain: "...not my will, but thine, be done." (Lk. 22:42)

But let us turn our thoughts back to His Incarnation. In light of our understanding of what will come at the Last Supper, at Gethsemane and at Golgotha, His words at the outset of His life take on a more remarkable meaning – almost a battle cry of consecration – as He takes on a human body prepared for Him: "Lo, I have come to do thy will, O God." This fiat of the Unborn Christ is both a consecration and proclamation of His mission on earth. This should be the essence of every Christian life as well.

A Communion of Two Fiats

Thankfully, this disposition of the Son as he came into the world was met in kind by the trusting disposition of His mother. "Behold, I am the handmaid of the Lord; let it be to me according to your word."(Lk 1:38) We see here a perfect match, a heart to heart accord, a meeting of minds, a predestined partnership between Son and Mother, between Almighty God and weak humanity. Not only did God love us first, but He first willed His own Incarnation. Mary's response: complete cooperation. Pope Pius XII quotes these two "fiats" together in one of his encyclical letters, placing Mary's chronologically first and then Christ's second, in conjunction with His acceptance of the Body given Him.[24]

Mary's actual words to Gabriel are like words of consecration: offering herself as Mother to the Son of God and an "offering" of her very body as a dwelling place for the body of the Unborn Son of God. As she offers herself and her body to God's service, so does her Son, the lesser precedes the greater One, as though to prefigure and anticipate Him. By preceding His redemptive consecration with her own modest maternal consecration, she sets the stage for what will be the most extraordinary relationship in all of history. Then from within her body He offers His own; it was the best thing that could have happened.

And so this launching of the Incarnation Mission from the womb of Mary got off to a great start! God's Plan was right on course, for this the turning point of human history and the starting point of the Savior's life. Divine Love was met with the best of humanity's love; God's Son was cherished by the most tender-hearted of mothers. And for the next nine months she would be His world, her body His little kingdom.

CHAPTER ONE ENDNOTES

1. Rev. L. C. Fillion, S.S., *The Life Of Christ*, trans. Rev. Newton Thompson, S.T.D. (St. Louis, MO: B. Herder Book Co., 1940), 256.
2. Rev. Frederick W. Faber, C. Orat., D.D., *Bethlehem* (Baltimore, MD: John Murphy & Co.), 62-63.
3. IBID., p.67.
4. Harriet Beecher Stowe, *Footsteps of the Master* (New York: J. B. Ford & Co., 1877), 72.
5. St. Thomas Aquinas, O.P., *Summa Theologica*, III, Question 33, Articles 1 and 4.
6. "Womb" is a general word given to the organ known as the uterus. The two fallopian tubes – also called in medical terms uterine tubes – extend from the uterus to the two ovaries and are associated with the uterus. The terms "womb" and "uterus" have long been used interchangeably. It has been a common practice also for people to speak of the womb as the place where conception (that is fertilization) and implantation occur and where the baby develops and grows for nine months. There is no contradiction between our present medical knowledge and Gabriel's statement to Mary that "...you will conceive in your womb and bear a son.. ." (Lk.1:31) because the term "womb" encompasses the uterus along with the uterine tubes. Further, prior to the early 1500s, the anatomical distinction between these parts had not yet been made.
7. Rev. Frederick W. Faber, C. Orat., D.D., *The Blessed Sacrament* (Baltimore, MD: John Murphy Company, circa 1855), 445.
8. Faber, *Bethlehem*, op. cit., pp.69-70.
9. St. Bonaventure, O.F.M., *Meditations On The Life Of Christ*, trans. Sister M. Emmanuel, O.S.B. (St. Louis, MO: B. Herder Book Co., 1934), 16.
10. *Catechism Of The Council Of Trent For Parish Priests*, trans. John A. McHugh, O.P., and Charles J. Callan, O.P. (New York: Joseph F. Wagner, Inc., 1934), 48.
11. Frank J. Sheed, *Theology And Sanity* (New York: Sheed And Ward, Inc., 1947), 172.
12. Jack Hayford, *The Mary Miracle* (Ventura, CA: Regal Books, 1994), 45,37.
13. Venerable Mary of Agreda, O.S.C., *Mystical City Of God*, Vol. II, trans. Fiscar Marison (Albuquerque, NM: Corcoran Publishing Co., 1902), 110-111, 116.
14. C. S. Lewis, *Mere Christianity* (New York: Simon & Schuster, 1996), 156.
15. In the foregoing quote from Heb.10.5-7, verses 6-8 of Psalm 40 are quoted as translated in the Greek Septuagint Bible. The Hebrew trans-

lation of Psalm 40, which is not quoted in this New Testament Book of Hebrews, would have read a bit differently; "...thou hast opened my ears. .." instead of the Greek "a body hast thou prepared for me..."

16. Pope Paul VI, *Devotion To The Blessed Virgin Mary*, trans. Vatican (Boston: Daughters of St. Paul, 1974), #20, 19.
17. St. Ignatius of Loyola, S.J., *Spiritual Exercises Of St. Ignatius* (New York: Frederick Pustet & Co., 1914), Part I, 2nd Week, 233-234.
18. F. F. Bruce et al., ed., *The International Bible Commentary* (Grand Rapids, MI: Zondervan Publishing House, 1986), 1524.
19. Blessed Columba Marmion, O.S.B., *Christ The Ideal Of The Monk*, 8th Edition, trans. by a nun of Tyburn Convent (St. Louis, MO: B. Herder Book Co., 1926), 109.
20. John Calvin, *Institutes of the Christian Religion*, Vol. I, trans. John Allen (Philadelphia, PA: Presbyterian Board of Christian Education, 1936), 527.
21. William M. Thompson, ed., *Berulle And The French School*, Selected Writings, trans. Lowell M. Glendon, S.S. (Mahwah, NJ: Paulist Press, 1989), 161, quoting Pierre De Berulle, *The Life Of Jesus.*
22. John Saward, *The Mysteries Of March* (Washington: The Catholic University of America Press, 1990), 21-22, quoting Hans Urs von Balthasar, *Der antiromische Affekt: Wie lasst sich das Papsttum in der Gesamtkirche integrieren* (Freiburg, 1974) 115.
23. Msgr. Robert Hugh Benson, *Christ In The Church*, 2nd Edition (St. Louis, MO: B. Herder, 1913), 8-9.
24. Pope Pius XII, "*On Devotion To The Sacred Heart Of Jesus*" (*Haurietis Aquas*), 1956, Heart Of The Saviour, ed. Josef Stierli, trans. Paul Andrew, S.J., (New York: Herder And Herder, 1958), 233.

2

Journey to the Hill Country of Judea

In those days Mary arose and went with haste into the hill country, to a city of Judah.
Luke 1:39

In the scriptures Mary is a person of action but not frivolity; she does not pursue activity for its own sake. Rather she acts with God at His prompt and pace. Why did Mary decide to go to the home of Elizabeth? Undoubtedly the Holy Spirit, who had come upon her (Lk 1:35), unfolded the reason for the angel's reference to Elizabeth's pregnancy. Her state, as she considered what she should do was described by St. Peter Julian Eymard:

> The Word was in Mary's womb. He inspired His Mother to visit Elizabeth; Mary carried to John his Master and King. John could not come, for his mother was too old to undertake that journey; Jesus Christ went to him. He did the same for us: we could not go to God; God came to us."[1]

Discerning the existence of some holy bond between the miraculous Divine intervention in her own life and a similar intervention in Elizabeth's life, or more specifically a direct connection between her son and Elizabeth's, she felt strongly that it was her duty to go and search out the possible significance of such a relationship and to even assist in furthering it. It is generally assumed that Mary had no intention of revealing to Elizabeth (or Zachariah, her husband) the miraculous pregnancy she carried, at least until God clearly showed her that she should. There is no doubt that she felt compelled to go and do God's Will.[2]

That she left "with haste" does not necessarily mean within minutes or hours. The Gospels are somewhat ambiguous about the time frames – departure, arrival and duration – of the journeys and visits that occurred during Mary's nine month pregnancy. For the sake of this reflection, we interpret "went with haste" as most likely meaning she left within a day or two, or at least within the week, for Mary was a practical and down to earth young woman who would have made appropriate arrangements before departing on this journey.

Mary set out on her three to four day journey. We are not told whether relatives or friends accompanied her.[3] Perhaps she traveled with a caravan heading towards Jerusalem. But if she was traveling in a group for all or part of the journey, we will assume that she was not doing a lot of talking. Rather she had hours upon hours to ponder in her heart all that had happened to her and the message that had been delivered to her. In the quiet of her thoughts and prayers a stream of realization flowed swiftly, carrying her along, and almost overflowing its banks. Father Faber presents the scene: "Like a new pulse of impetuous gladness, the Babe in Mary's Bosom drives her forth. With swift step, as if the precipitate gracefulness of her walk were the outward sign of her inward joy, and she were beating time with her body to the music that was so jubilant within...."[4]

This is the first Christian missionary journey undertaken for the sake of the Gospel of Jesus Christ! Unborn Jesus initiates it, He and his mother go out prefiguring the missionary journeys initiated by Jesus, when He sent out first the twelve apostles and then the seventy disciples two by two (Mk 6:7 and Lk 10:1). Christians traveling on mission, in pairs, had not only a spiritual and psychological purpose, but also an ecclesiastical one; the two together are in communion one with the other, experiencing Christ's power acting through them and their different gifts and talents. In the case of pregnant Mary, here we have the quintessential communion, the epitome of communion with Christ. Two lives intertwine in the messianic mission and the world's greatest love.

Most likely Mary welcomed these three or four days of traveling as it afforded her a great deal of time to reflect and pray and to sort out in her own mind what had happened, what had been said, and so on. Complementing those gifts she had received from the Holy Spirit were common sense which kept her from becoming flustered or rash and her accrued wisdom – much advanced for her age – which held her back from imprudent speculations. She trusted that God would continue to guide her along this untraveled path and explain to her in appropriate incremental measures the mystery she had entered. Underlying all her thoughts was a poignant sense of duty and mission – the messianic mission. As Cardinal Berulle explains, her unique role was underway:

> The Virgin is involved with Jesus and she is the only one in the whole world involved with Jesus. Thus she is the only one in the whole world adoring the mystery of the Incarnation, which was brought about on earth for the earth but unknown to the earth. She is the only one adoring Jesus. The more that she is the only one captivated by such a great subject, the greater is her involvement. She is devoted to it with all her faculties. All her senses are brought to bear on it, for it is a tangible mystery and tangible within her. All her senses should pay homage to her God made tangible for human nature. Her whole mind is concentrated on it. And the Spirit of Jesus, which enlivens this little divinized body, enlivens the spirit and body of the Virgin as well, through grace, love and a holy, gentle influence.[5]

Before considering Mary's reaction to her situation and her reflections upon Gabriel's message, let us delve a bit deeper into this mystery of the Incarnation.

The Redemptive Pregnancy: A Hidden Spiritual Reality

Consider for a moment some of the parables or images Jesus used in describing the kingdom of heaven to help us appreciate the mystery of His nine months in the womb. For example, in Matthew 13:

> The kingdom of heaven is like a grain of mustard seed which a man took and sowed in his field; it is the smallest of all seeds, but when it has grown it is the greatest of shrubs and becomes a tree...
>
> The kingdom of heaven is like leaven which a woman took and hid in three measures of meal...
>
> The kingdom of heaven is like treasure hidden in a field...

> ...the kingdom of heaven is like a merchant in search of fine pearls, who, on finding one pearl of great value, went and sold all that he had and bought it.

These parables emphasize the hidden quality of the kingdom of God as unseen and unknown. This is precisely the dominant quality of Unborn Jesus: hidden, unseen, unknown and unborn. He is the tiniest seed growing in secret, the leaven acting upon the body within which it is placed, the hidden treasure and valuable pearl which inspired decisive acts by those who discovered it.

In the preceding quote the great French spiritual writer Berulle refers to "the mystery of the Incarnation". Both Jesus and St. Paul had similarly used the word "mystery" in related contexts as well:

> And he said unto them, "Unto you it is given to know the mystery of the kingdom of God" Mk 4:11 (KJV).

> Withal praying also for us, that God would open unto us a door of utterance, to speak the mystery of Christ Col 4:3 (KJV).

Now when Jesus, Paul or Berulle use the term "mystery", what are they suggesting? They refer to profound realities that are spiritual and hidden but which have been revealed by the Holy Spirit (see Paul's comments: I Cor:2.6-13). "Mystery" understood in this sense is a powerful and essential biblical concept. But today people often associate mystery with suspense stories, plot twists, surprise endings or guessing a concealed identity. Yet because something is a mystery doesn't make it myth or fiction. And because something is spiritual doesn't make it unreal. For indeed God is Spirit and He created the physical world we live in, from nothing. So spiritual reality provides the foundation for all physical reality. The tiny body of Jesus in the womb of Mary is a physical reality. But both preceding and surrounding this reality are numerous spiritual realities, and herein lies one of the greatest mysteries of the Christian faith.

The term "mystical" has the same root word as "mystery" and seems to have better retained the biblical sense of the word in contemporary use.[6] Over the centuries Christians have come to appreciate this word because it unites together the concepts of "mystery" and "spiritual reality" as they are to be experienced by the individual Christian. (At the end of this chapter we will come back to this point.)

We can describe the relationship between Unborn Jesus and His mother as being primarily mystical in nature. His manner of influencing, inspiring, and consoling her, whether directly or indirectly, was hidden from all people. But it was more than a physical reality; it was, first and foremost, a potent spiritual reality which she experienced in wonderment. Unborn Jesus, like the mustard seed or leaven, was active and dynamic within His mother's womb. And His mother recognized His infinite "value", or rather how far beyond a mere treasure or "pearl of great value" He was. So she who had conceived by the Spirit of God was also by that same Spirit enlightened regarding this unique "mystical" relationship.

Mary Reflects on All That Has Occurred Thus Far

Since the mother of Jesus is the original source for much that scripture relates about Unborn Jesus, we need to pause and consider how Mary is reacting to these momentous events. But before we consider her thoughts in more detail, we must note that thought process and subject matter have changed from then to our own day.

Two thousand years after Christ, memories are vast warehouses of minutiae: telephone numbers, the call letters of radio stations, song lyrics, batting averages, grocery prices, information obtained from the newspaper, radio, television, internet, or study, international facts, news, and scientific data: a virtual ocean of things we never even intended to remember. Much of this "stuff" we learn without deliberate intention because of the constant and endless stream of information that we must face each day. Yet our memories sort out all of this material with precision and skill beyond comprehension.

The human memory, which we tend to take for granted, is a marvelous faculty of the soul and a true source of formative insightfulness for each person. In the book *Daily Life in the Time of Jesus*, Henri Daniel-Rops observes:

> Our memories have become anemic and impotent; our improvising abilities are far more didactic than poetic. This was not at all the case in Israel, nor indeed among the other Eastern nations. Thought was handed on, handed down in the most lasting and permanent manner, very largely by the spoken word; and this, of course, necessarily affected the spoken word, giving it some very particular char-

> acteristics.....since all the texts that were learnt by heart were taken from the Scriptures, the learner's mind was stored with biblical facts, sentences and figures, which explains the innumerable scriptural echoes that were to be heard in the speech of the Jewish men and women of that time....It must be emphasized that this systematic training of the memory was not only for specialists....children were brought up to learn by rote from the earliest age.[7]

In rural Galilee several thousand years ago, the people had little to remember besides religious and historical lore and local-familial information. We are not here belittling them. On the contrary, not only were their minds as sharp and as capable as ours, but they were focused on fewer but select things. Day to day details such as the names and ages of a distant cousin's family members would be much more naturally remembered than in today's world. While the intellectual stimulation and pursuits of those living two thousand years ago were far different from those of today, and while we might call them, by today's standards, "technologically deficient," we would be sadly mistaken if we thought them to be in any way intellectually deficient.

Given these different environments and mental aptitudes, we can assume that the words spoken to Mary captivated her more than a similar experience would captivate one of our contemporaries. Mary's recollection of the wording would be much more accurate than ours. Daily encounters with people took the place of our newspapers, books, tapes, movies, radio, television, computers and so on. Thousands of words were not being aimed at her every minute and hour of every day. Mary's attentive mind was free to remember and contemplate the relatively short message given her by the Archangel Gabriel.

". . .and you shall call His name Jesus"

From a psychological perspective, we must assume that one word of the angel's message was imprinted upon her very soul as if by a burning coal – the name of her baby, the name of God's baby: Jesus. How many thousands of times did she whisper this name softly to herself or reverently call it to mind as her steps and thoughts carried her (and her newly conceived Son) across the future missionary territory of Galilee and Judea? And yet neither Mary nor even the angel had given the Child this Name. "That Name, 'which is above all names,' was given by God Himself (Phil

2:9); and it was eternally His. Just as He was eternally begotten of His Father, so He was eternally named by His Father.....The second Person of the Blessed Trinity had ever been Jesus, the Savior." [8]

The journey would have been punctuated by Mary's calm, simple repetition of this singular Name; and in her devotion to this Name, the Church's own devotion to the Holy Name of Jesus began. Mary would have treasured this Name and become enamored by it very quickly. Knowing the meaning of the Name God had chosen – "Yahweh is Salvation" – Mary knew the great mission of her Son. Repeating the Name – and especially audibly hearing it pronounced – would have brought joy to her soul. Maternal joy yes, but more than that: joy as the Lord's faithful handmaid, and joy as a witness to the fulfillment of God's promises. "O Lord, our Lord, how majestic is thy name in all the earth"! (Psalm 8:1) No doubt it would be verses and biblical passages such as this one that a devout Israelite like Mary would call to mind as she reflected on her situation.

But, another "word" also must have gripped her soul with weeping joy. As Mother Mary Potter puts it: "....He spoke a voiceless word, and that word was 'Mother'..."[9] Though the angel had not used this "word", this was the reality of her situation. She discovered her motherhood by contemplating the baby within her – her baby.

Her thoughts probably were directed to other biblical mothers who conceived in miraculous fashion: Sarah, Abraham's wife, who at the age of ninety (Gen 17:1, 17:17, 18:14) gave birth to her only son Isaac; the mother of Samson to whom an angel had appeared to announce the upcoming birth of a special child; the wealthy Shunammite woman who conceived a son as the prophet Elisha had promised (2 Kings 4:12-17); and finally Hannah, Samuel's mother, who received an indication from Eli the priest that she would bear a son, and then offered her son for service in the temple. Hannah's words of thanksgiving and worship are preserved in the scriptures as a canticle with which Mary was very familiar.[10]

Mary surely would have reflected upon these four barren women to whom God had promised sons. But all of these women conceived as a result of natural relations with their husbands. Mary would quickly realize that her situation was different in many respects. She was *not* barren. She was *not* elderly. She did *not* conceive through natural relations with Joseph. The content of the angel's message was very different, too. A prophesy surpassing all others had been given about the child. The angel explained how this conception would occur and then gave Mary additional instruction and teaching. As Mary walked the road south towards Judea she could not have helped but marvel at the unparalleled circumstances of the situation she was in. Yet she believed.

As she reconsidered the words spoken by the angel, her mind tried to come to terms with their meaning: "...the Lord God will give to Him the throne of His father David, and He will reign over the house of Jacob for ever; and of His kingdom there will be no end" (Lk 1:32-33).

Her son was the Messiah! What other explanation could possibly make any sense? She is the first Saint of the Incarnation, called and destined to love the Son of God and to collaborate with Him in every aspect of His Incarnation mission. From Gabriel's announcement Mary knew that Jesus was King and had come to establish His kingdom on earth. She was merely His handmaid, but would do all she could to help bring this kingdom into being according to God's Will. For now she could pray for the coming of the kingdom, perhaps in words not so very different from: "Father God in Heaven, Thy Kingdom come, Thy Will be done, on earth as it is in Heaven."

For those of us today who are devoted to this Unborn Jesus, it is important to see that, based on Gabriel's incarnation message quoted above, Unborn Jesus is a King intent upon taking possession of His Kingdom and establishing His reign. But what of the angel's other words? What did Mary make of them?

> He will be great, and will be called the Son of the Most High (Lk 1:32).

> The Holy Spirit will come upon you, and the power of the Most High will overshadow you; therefore the child to be born will be called holy, the Son of God (Lk 1:35).

The Holy Spirit had already overshadowed her; her being had been bathed in the light of grace and she believed she had already conceived.

Because she had a simple and pure faith, her tendency would be to accept everything the angel said to her. Yet the intellect got dizzy as it scaled upward towards the lofty meaning of each word and phrase uttered. Not once, but twice, the angel had referred to her son as God's Son. While her heart leapt to the plain meaning of the words, her mind stood still in awe of them. Joy not to be defined invaded every pore, every cell, every region of her being.

Some might argue that Mary could not have understood what these words meant, nor would she understand them to mean what we Christians now understand them to mean: "...God from God, light from light, true God from true God, begotten not made, one in being with the Father..." (As the Nicean Creed states.) A Catholic Biblical scholar states:

> Mary now knew the divine purpose – but did she understand it? Above all, did she realize that the child to be born of her would be divine? If we look to the essentials of Luke's narrative we find that his attention first bears on the child whose birth he announces, then on the motherhood of Mary and lastly on the manner of her maternity. In other words, the central fact, and the source of the others, is the Incarnation, and this, by definition, means that God became Man. It forms the kernel of the angel's message and if Mary had not grasped this she had not really understood the message. But, according to the principles of the literary form in question, she ought to have understood the message before the departure of the angel, and Luke's treatment of the matter implied that she had. We may maintain, therefore, not gratuitously but with sound reason, that at the moment of the Incarnation, Mary knew that the child then and there conceived in her womb was divine. This, however, is not to claim that she was fully enlightened (cf. 2:50; 2:19,51); and we are told that her *Fiat* was essentially an act of faith (1:45) – which included, in its object, the divinity of Christ, but seen in the darkness that is a necessary feature of faith.[11]

Mary received the gospel message from an angel, and she had grasped its essence. She accepted it, and as the Fathers of the Church have pointed out, she believed even before she conceived, or rather, she conceived in her heart before conceiving in her womb.[12] She not only has the proper missionary spirit but she knows what she is about. It is not her journey; it is the Messiah's Mission!

As we picture Mary traversing the countryside towards her inspired destination, she is the simplest of vessels carrying the most precious of contents. Indeed, there is in the Old Testament a remarkable prefigurement of this journey and the three month visit which is about to take place. We read in the second book of Samuel (6:1-13) of the Ark of the Covenant being brought to the home of Obededom where it remains for three months.[13]

Unborn Jesus in Perspective

In the first few days of a pregnancy there is life wrapped in mystery. Who knows of its presence? In the first few days of a new human life only God knows. "In those days", when Mary leaves Nazareth for Judea, that is in the first few days of Jesus' human life, Embryonic Jesus is extremely tiny in physical size. He is of little account. What can we learn from Him in such a minute state of existence? In the twelfth century St. Bernard shed some light on this question: "How could he have shown his mercy more clearly than by taking on himself our condition? For our sake the Word of God became as grass....The incarnation teaches us how much God cares for us and what he thinks and feels about us...The smaller he became through his human nature the greater was his goodness; the more he lowered himself for me, the dearer he is to me."[14]

The less He resembles God or man, the more He seems to be giving of Himself to me! In the embryonic state He is at His least, but He is at His least for me! This biological perspective gives new meaning to St. Paul's famous summation about our Lord's Incarnation: "...though he was in the form of God, did not count equality with God a thing to be grasped, but emptied himself...." (Phil 2:6-7). And in becoming human in this manner, Jesus as embryo doesn't even look like a human and becomes despised by many others, as are many human embryos today. (He also receives the same pejorative epithets hurled disrespectfully at Him – 'a mere collection of cells', 'potential life', a speck of dust – that are irresponsibly tossed at others now in that state of human existence.)

Perhaps His smallness is like the poor widow who put two copper coins in the Temple treasury (Mk 12:41-44). She is wretched in her poverty, but for that very reason she gives more! The Embryonic Jesus blessed our world in ways we will never fathom and to degrees we could never imagine.

We typically do not look at the Incarnation in terms of the stages of our Lord's human development. Yet we must cherish Jesus Christ and adore Him in every human stage of His development, seeing in each stage of His growth yet another way that He reaches out to us, communicating through this way and that His solidarity with humanity, His redemptive solution for each individual's malaise and His intimate love for every person. Mary knew that God loved her tiny unborn child–through every stage of his precious life–with an immensely tender love. So should every mother know this same truth about her unborn child!

From the earliest days of His human existence Unborn Jesus set out to win His mother's heart. In fact, every unborn child on a primitive natural level has this same objective. Most succeed. But it is more than simply a survival mechanism. Love not only makes the world go 'round but it also eases mother and child through nine 'challenging' months of pregnancy! Love is to persons what 'meaning' is to life. When it comes to a mother and her unborn child both are imperative. Tragically, modern medicine has perverted this truth by severing these intimately connected realities from each other, so that [unborn] human life is no longer held sacred and love for [unborn] children is no longer deemed natural or necessary.

The mother, conscious of God's steadfast love and holy esteem for her unborn child, strives daily to share in the divine attitude towards the unseen, unknown child, and as the months pass she is drawn into the sacredness of her relationship and responsibility to her unborn child. (And of course, with the birth comes a rush of natural human love and corresponding emotions to support the mother in her role.) Thankfully, Unborn Jesus and His mother provide the world with the original Christian model for this most basic human relationship. In this we can find tremendous supernatural encouragement and hope for the future.

"I Am the Way. . . ." (Jn 14:6)

Decades later, the Son of God called Himself "the Way" and He truly is that! After ascending into heaven He also called Himself "the Alpha and the Omega" (Rev 1:8,22:13). This title clearly shows His eternal identity especially as it relates to our human history. But He is also the Alpha not only through His initial role in creation, but in His creation of each individual life, and the Omega for each person's life through His role as the Crucified and resurrected King.

In 1979, in his book *Aborting America* Dr. Bernard Nathanson introduced the designation 'alpha' as a neutral term for referring to the unborn baby in the womb.[15] Ironically Jesus Christ had already claimed Alpha as His own title. A further way of understanding Jesus as Alpha, following Dr. Nathanson's thinking, is as a prototype for all unborn babies. "He blazed a trail, and if we follow it, life and death are made holy and take on a new meaning."[16]

We find in the New Testament letter to the Hebrews some sign posts which point to the reality and identity of Jesus Who is "The Way". Let's look at some of the titles given to the Son of God in Hebrews, considering these as they might relate specifically to Unborn Jesus Who is the incipient Way.

The Pioneer of (Our) Salvation	Heb 2:10
The Pioneer and Perfecter of Our Faith	Heb 12:2
A Forerunner on Our Behalf	Heb 6:20
A High Priest For Ever (after the Order of Melchizedek)	Heb 6:20
The First-Born	Heb 1:6
The Heir of All Things	Heb 1:2
The Same Yesterday and Today and For Ever	Heb13:8

From His first moment in the womb Unborn Jesus became the pioneer of our salvation and faith, as a forerunner perfecting a way for us to live and believe. Unborn Jesus is the singular pioneer for every human life. As His mother Mary's footsteps trace in history's dust transitory footprints meandering their way towards the hill country of Judea, His inaudible and invisible footsteps begin the greatest missionary and pioneering adventure that the world will ever witness! He is on a mission and as the first-born heir of all things He is interested in finding all the lost sheep of this world and providing them with a reliable leader and path to follow. But He also comes as Priest intent upon offering Himself when His earthly sojourn comes to an end. In His first days of earthly human existence He is no less the pioneer or Priest than He will be thirty-three years hence, for He is the same yesterday and today and for ever!

Note that the seven titles listed above relate to time. For an unborn child time is a meaningless concept because the unborn child, while experiencing things within the womb – movements and sensations, noises and tastes – does not have a standard of time for relating the duration of such experiences. And yet, perhaps there is one appropriate though distant "standard" by which the unborn child can measure experience – eternity. For every unborn child is left on eternity's doorstep, alone within a womb. Nameless, faceless, unknown, uncounted, perhaps unwanted, and to many apparently unreal! Not the most notable of beginnings.

From the very heart and center of eternity comes Unborn Jesus our one and only leader. His mission in the Incarnation is like one drawn out loving embrace by the eternal God. And from these hidden human beginnings within a womb He demonstrates a new way of existing in relation to God and creation. His life will be punctuated by key historical and redemptive bodily events: incarnation/conception, birth, crucifixion, resurrection and ascension. Through baptism the Christian is joined to the Body of Christ and participates in these events in a mystical sense. St. Paul made reference to this mystery of faith: "Do you not know that all of us who have been baptized into Christ Jesus were baptized into his death?....For if we have been united to him in a death like his, we shall certainly be united with him in a resurrection like his"(Rom 6:3,5).

But Christ the Omega of our lives is also the Alpha of our lives. His redemptive actions become accessible to us through baptism and grace. St. Leo the Great (died 461 A.D.) explained that: "....the birthday of the Head is the birthday of the Body....the entire body of the faithful, born in the baptismal font, is born with Christ in His nativity, just as all are crucified with Him in His passion, raised again in His resurrection, and set at the Father's right hand in His ascension."[17]

We who are mystically joined to Christ through our baptism follow behind Him, our Head, as a thread follows behind the needle which is sewing together that which was apart.[18] Our pioneer leader – the pioneer of our faith and salvation – is joining in Himself the divine life with our human life, heaven with earth, eternity with our temporal existence. In baptism we die with Christ and are raised with Christ, but also we are conceived with Christ and born with Christ!

Pulling all of this together is the fact that Jesus is a Pioneer in how He loved God and people. His heartbeat would set a new spiritual standard, like a tuning fork or the central clock by which all others are set. His priestly Heart, model for all human hearts, the One that set them all in motion and draws them all heavenward, even now quickly within His mother's womb beats, beats, beats for Love.

The Church, the Mystical Body of Christ Is Formed

The archangel Gabriel also had spoken to Mary of the kingship of her Son. This is a concept that Mary could not have understood fully, yet would have appreciated nonetheless. Mary would not have perceived the meaning of the Church in the terminology that St. Paul and others would later use to explain it. St. Paul took the reference by Jesus many years later to His Body being a temple, and developed the teaching concerning the identity of the Church as in fact "the Body of Christ". For example, Paul said that baptized Christians "are the body of Christ and individually members of it" (I Cor 12:27) and that Jesus Christ "is the head of the body, the church..." (Col 1:18). So, at the one cell stage of the formation of the physical Body of Jesus Christ, we also acknowledge the formation of the spiritual (mystical) Body of Christ, that is, the Church. Theologian Karl Adam explains: "It is clear therefore, in the light of the redemption, that the Church did not come into being only when Peter and John and Paul became believers. It became objectively existent when the divine Word united His nature with human nature in the unity of His person. The Incarnation is for Christians the foundation and planting of that new communion which we call the Church. The Body of Christ and the Kingdom of God came into being as objective reality at the moment when the Word was made flesh."[19]

In this same discussion, Adam also refers to the Church at this initial point as "an organic community". Another spiritual writer puts it this way: "At the same moment and by the same act there came into existence the Redeemer and the redeemed."[20]

This should not be surprising given the profound identification developed in the letters of St. Paul between Christ and the Body of Christ (the Church). We might pause here for a moment to marvel at the full beauty and majesty of the Incarnation Mission, especially at that one cell stage of the bodily existence of Jesus Christ. In the last chapter we said that the first cell of the Body of Unborn Jesus was the cornerstone of His physical body. But it is also the cornerstone of His Mystical Body, the Church.

Since Christ came as Redeemer, we can best understand Him in terms of His relationships to others. At the dawning of His physical earthly life we also witness the dawning of our redemption. And we are represented here by one humble human being – the young handmaiden, Mary of Nazareth. Hence we can say that Mary is the first member of the Mystical Body of Christ, the Church, at its inception. Thankfully, she accepted the gospel as proclaimed to her by God's angelic evangelist Gabriel. She then proceeded to act on behalf of the Church, to collaborate with and cooperate with and indeed to serve the Lord. So while the Church owes its very existence, identity and mission to Jesus Christ, its first member and exemplar is Mary in her capacity as mother to the Redeemer.

"For with God nothing will be impossible."

Finally, we return again to Mary and particularly her response to those final words spoken to her by the Archangel Gabriel. Every pregnant mother can use some encouraging words. This little tidbit of angelic wisdom is a quotable quote par excellence, "For with God nothing will be impossible"(cf. Gen 18:14). Here is the thought that Gabriel leaves with Mary, a piece of advice for the road. Certainly she must have called this phrase to mind repeatedly as she traveled towards the hill country. This sound angelic advice would serve her well in the months ahead.

Mary probably repeated this phrase for the rest of her life. One reason for assuming this is that our Lord seems to have borrowed this expression from his mother and "made it His own". The following are a few examples of this:

> But Jesus looked at them and said to them, "With men this is impossible, but with God all things are possible" Mt 19:26.

> And He said, "Abba, Father, all things are possible to Thee; remove this cup from me; yet not what I will, but what Thou wilt" Mk 14:36.[21]

In fact, Jesus seems to have taken this family saying and even turned it around a little bit as follows:

> And Jesus said to him, "If you can! All things are possible to him who believes" Mk 9:23.

Mary no doubt carefully considered all of the angel's words. She believed them and was even now acting upon them. They became for her a Credo, a germinating gospel around which her life would be lived.

Jesus Begins His Journey towards Humanity

No sooner did Christ become incarnate than He began seeking out the lost sheep of Israel, pioneering the way for our salvation. Conception normally occurs in the fallopian tube and this newly conceived Christ was journeying down that tube towards the uterus where His Body, a blastocyst, would implant for the remainder of the pregnancy. Yet the journey in search of hearts, like Elizabeth's (and unborn John's) and Zechariah's, was also underway and He was traveling to the outskirts of Jerusalem now on His first missionary journey. Since the typical journey down the fallopian tube takes four to seven days, and the journey from Nazareth to Judea (probably the town of Ain-Karim) takes three to four days, it may have happened that both these initial journeys began and/or ended at approximately the same time. Inasmuch as Mary represents the people and nation of Israel, the journey of Unborn Jesus within her can also represent the outward journey, both journeys being carried out in accordance with the Father's will.

CHAPTER TWO ENDNOTES

1. St. Peter Julian Eymard, S.S.S. *The Real Presence – Eucharistic Meditations* (New York, NY: The Sentinel Press, 1938), 297-298.
2. "We can feel the rush of warmth and kindness, the sudden urgency of love that sent that girl hurrying over the hills. 'Those days' in which she rose on that impulse were the days in which Christ was being formed in her, the impulse was His impulse." See Caryll Houselander, *The Reed of God* (Westminster, MD: Christian Classics, Inc., 1990), 32.
3. The New Testament does not mention that anyone traveled with Mary, nor does it state that she traveled alone. Several mystics state that Joseph accompanied her to the home of Elizabeth and Zechariah, that he remained there about three days or so and then he returned alone to Nazareth. See Venerable Mary of Agreda, O.S.C., *Mystical City of God,* Vol. II, trans. Fiscar Marison (Albuquerque, NM: Corcoran Publishing Co., 1902), 167-168. See Venerable Anne Catherine Emmerich, O.S.A., *The Life of the Blessed Virgin Mary,* trans. Sir Michael Palairet (Rockford, IL: Tan Books and Publishers, Inc., 1970), 146.
4. Rev. Frederick W. Faber, C.Orat., D.D., *Bethlehem* (Baltimore, MD: John Murphy & Co.), 81.
5. William M. Thompson, ed., *Berulle And The French School,* Selected Writings, trans. Lowell M. Glendon, S.S. (Mahwah, NJ: Paulist Press, 1989), 164.
6. "The word mystical and the word mystery (which is the reality behind the notion of sacrament) are related. The word mystery in the bible designates the saving plan of God, the blueprint of salvation history, the designs of His will. Later, it came to designate the sacramental rights, not in the sense that these are to remain hidden or mysterious, but in that through them we are assimilated into the mystery or plan of God in Christ: the one paschal mystery. The adjective mystical (which originally meant only "hidden" or "secret" with out any religious connotation) came to characterize the sacramental experience of the mystery or plan of God into which we are assimilated by sacramental celebration. Accordingly, mystical also designated that interpretation of Scripture and that proclamation of the Word which was centered on the one paschal mystery: the salvific power of the death and resurrection of Christ." Cardinal William Baum, "Address to the Federation of Catholic Scholars." L'Osservatore Romano (Vatican City), December 7, 1978, p. 6. For an explanation regarding the term Mystical Body of Christ, see section # 60-66 of Pope Pius XII's Encyclical *Mystici Corporis Christi.* .

7. Henri Daniel-Rops, *Daily Life In The Time Of Jesus* trans. Patrick O'Brian (New York, NY: Hawthorn Books, Inc., 1962), 309, 311.
8. Mother St. Paul, *Nativitas Christi* (London: Longmans, Green and Co. Ltd., 1937), 31...
9. Mother Mary Potter, *The Path of Mary*, 6th edition (Chicago, IL: Little Company of Mary, 1878), 53.
10. Some of the sentiments from Hannah's canticle are later echoed in Mary's. See I Sam.2.1-8.
11. Rev. Reginald C. Fuller et al., ed., *A New Catholic Commentary on Holy Scripture*, revised (London: Thomas Nelson and Sons Ltd., 1975), 997
12. St.Leo the Great (Pope 440-461 A.D.), *Sermo 1 in Nativitate Domini*, 2.3: PL 54, 191-192.
13. The similarities between the ancient Ark of the Covenant and Mary the Ark of the "New" Covenant are numerous. Both were overshadowed by the Spirit of God. Obededom's house was in the same vicinity as the home of Zechariah and Elizabeth. Both visits lasted about three months. David danced with merriment before the ancient Ark and unborn John leaped with joy before Mary (who carried Unborn Jesus). David asked "How can the ark of the Lord come to me?" and Elizabeth exclaimed "... why is this granted me, that the mother of my Lord should come to me?" Other parallels exist as well.
14. St. Bernard, O. Cist., *Sermo 1, in Ephiphania Domini*, 1-2: PL 133. 141-143, *In Christian Prayer: The Liturgy Of The Hours* (Boston, MA: Daughters of St. Paul, 1976), 1655.
15. Bernard N. Nathanson, M.D., *Aborting America (New York: Doubleday* & Co,, 1979) 179.
16. Vatican II, *Gaudium et Spes* 22, in *Documents of Vatican II,* Rev. Walter M. Abbott, S.J. et al., ed., (New York: America Press, 1966), 221.
17. St. Leo the Great, *Sermon 26, 2 on the Feast of the Nativity*, PL 54, 213..
18. This needle and thread image is an imperfect one. But it does illustrate in two ways how Christ acts in our regard. First, like the Divine Physician he treats the wound of sin by cleansing it in the baptismal waters and then stitching it back together. Secondly, He does not sew a new "unshrunk cloth on an old garment" for fear that such a new "patch tears away from the (old) garment" (Mt.9.16). Rather, He first takes on the human condition, then as Son of Man joins Himself to us, then we become new in Christ.
19. Karl Adam, *The Spirit of Catholicism*, trans. Justin McCann, O.S.B. (Garden City, New York: Doubleday & Company, Inc., 1954), 35-36.
20. Martin Jenneskens, *The Eucharist and Life*, trans. Gregory G. Rybrook (Paterson, N.J.: St. Anthony Guild Press, 1948), 36-37

21. The tenderness and meekness of this prayer, uttered by Jesus the night before His death, is all the more striking as He might be paraphrasing words that He learned from His mother as a little boy.

3

Exchange of Prophetic Greetings

As Mary neared her journey's end, ascending winding paths into the hill country towards the home of her cousin, her delight and expectation heightened. In contrast, Elizabeth would have been in a more subdued frame of mind as she did not expect any visitors.

St. Luke relates that in the first months of her pregnancy Elizabeth "hid herself" (Lk 1:24); that is, kept to herself more than usual, spending more time in and around her home. Given her age, condition, and recent habits it seems likely that she would have been in her house as Mary approached and thus caught by surprise:

> . . . .and she entered the house of Zechariah and greeted Elizabeth. And when Elizabeth heard the greeting of Mary, the babe leaped in her womb; and Elizabeth was filled with the Holy Spirit and she exclaimed with a loud cry, "Blessed are you among women, and blessed is the fruit of your womb! And why is this granted me, that the mother of my Lord should come to me? For behold, when the voice of your greeting came to my ears, the babe in my womb leaped for joy. And blessed is she who believed that there would be a fulfillment of what was spoken to her from the Lord." And Mary said, "My soul magnifies the Lord" Lk 1:40-46.

This extraordinary meeting captures the meaning of the Incarnation in a unique way. This is the "inside story" so to speak. Just as invisible God became man to communicate with us, so in this meeting the invisible babies act to communicate with Elizabeth, Mary, you and me. To assist us in studying this first manifestation of the Incarnation of God, we will first list the separate acts in order of occurrence, and then examine each in greater depth.

1. Mary enters the house of Zechariah and Elizabeth
2. Mary greets Elizabeth
3. Unborn baby John leaps within his mother
4. Elizabeth is filled with the Holy Spirit
5. Elizabeth greets and blesses Mary, recounting John's joy
6. Mary responds to Elizabeth with her song of joyful praise.

1. Mary Enters the Home of Elizabeth

She had finally reached her destination after a three-or-four day journey; road weary perhaps, but probably energized by an unprecedented Messianic joy mingled with maternal expectation. This Messianic joy would be a hallmark of her pregnancy as she and others would savor the realization of God's cherished promises, the fulfillment of age old prophecies and the immediate tangible presence of God unborn. This young mother was ready for God, ready for the unexpected and something unexpected happened almost immediately.

2. Mary Greets Elizabeth

Mary's prayerful and quiet journey caused her to be intensely focused at the moment of her arrival, filled with good will and God within. Exactly what she said is unknown, but surely Mary's greeting was simple and joyful. Yet, though the words were ordinary, the context of their utterance was extraordinary. Remember Mary had undertaken a journey at the veiled suggestion of the Archangel Gabriel, acting as Messenger of Almighty God. Her sincere words of greeting were a heavenly key, carefully drawn out for the purposes of the Lord, unlocking Heaven's hidden vault, and so setting in motion a series of inspired events and multiple testimonies to the joy the Messiah brings.

3. Unborn Baby John "Leaps" Within His Mother

Initially the scene is commonplace. Two women – the older one visibly pregnant – meet in a quaint ordinary encounter. For the older woman's baby, it seems, just a typical day in the monotonous life of an "insignificant" unborn child. But now the scene descends into the uncharted amniotic waters of the womb. The secret life of the unborn infants and the hidden acts of the unseen God unfold unexpectedly. No human playwright created this scene: the Holy Spirit narrates this spiritual "ultrasound." John is every unborn child, symbolically the least of all people. God enters, like every unborn baby – unseen, unheard, unknown – to comfort and bless all unborn babies, all children, all adults, all of the least among us – everyone – to the last, to the least. The salvation of humanity is prefigured here.

Since salvation is personal, it begins with one person. The mystery of God's intervention in one's life is one of the greatest mysteries a person experiences, particularly as God acts first. [1] So here, before unborn John leaps for joy, there is "the cause".

Unborn Jesus, possibly less than a week old, though minuscule and voiceless, was not powerless. Though well less than one hundredth the size of unborn baby John, much less than one thousandth the size of Mary or Elizabeth, He is in control. As Mary spoke, He acted. Her voice became His vehicle, her greeting His instrument. As Father Faber wrote:

> Truly He is in haste to be about His Father's business. Truly He is an impatient conqueror, to be thus early beginning His conquests, and laying the foundations of His world-wide empire. He cannot bear to be in the world for even so short a while, but sin shall feel the weight of His unborn arm.....His first mission and ministry was in the womb, and the babe unborn the first conquest of His divine apostolate.....and the Unborn Child destroys the sin and abolishes the curse of the unborn child. [2]

This unborn encounter is not accidental. On the contrary, God planned the encounter. Recall that the angel Gabriel told Zechariah that John would "be filled with the Holy Spirit, even from his mother's womb"(Lk 1:15). These events, and the relationship between John and Jesus are indirectly alluded to by the prophet Malachi: "Behold, I send my messenger to prepare the way before me, and the Lord whom you seek will suddenly come to his temple......he will sit as a refiner and purifier of silver, and he will purify the sons of Levi and refine them like gold and silver, till they present right offerings to the Lord." (Mal 3:1,3).

Zechariah, the father of unborn John, was an Aaronic priest: hence, a "son of Levi", and thus John also was a "son of Levi". Zechariah was, at the time of this encounter, midway through his purifying penance, having lost the ability to speak after doubting the message of the

Archangel Gabriel (Lk 1:20). At the exact moment of Mary's greeting of Elizabeth, Unborn Jesus purifies the unborn prophet John with, what might be described as a baptism with the Holy Spirit (cf. Lk 1:15, Jn 1:33). This event then fulfils Gabriel's promise as well as Malachi's prophecy.

This extraordinary encounter shares many elements with baptism especially infant baptism.[3] Unborn John is immersed in the waters of the womb as Mary speaks her greeting – in a sense, Mary speaks "in the name of the Father and of the Son and of the Holy Spirit": the Father Who chose her, sent Gabriel to her and overshadowed her, the Son Whom she carries within and the Holy Spirit Who came upon her and by Whom she conceived. The Spirit descends upon the unborn infant John to fulfill the angel's promise: "...he will be filled with the Holy Spirit, even from his mother's womb" (Lk 1:15).

Remarkably, this is the first perceived act of Jesus recorded in the Gospel accounts after He comes into the world, although the first hidden act of Unborn Jesus was to offer Himself to His Father (see chapter I). Here His first evangelistic act, reaching out directly to humanity, is discovered. This act prefigures baptism and anticipates His final teaching, given as He was about to ascend into Heaven: "Go therefore and make disciples of all nations, baptizing them in the name of the Father and of the Son and of the Holy Spirit" (Mt 28:19). These two acts – one before birth and the other after death – seem to emphasize the importance of baptism.

Now the preaching of Jesus expanded upon the idea of baptism introducing the central role of the Holy Spirit. This flows very consistently out of: 1. the intrauterine "baptism" of John, and 2. the baptism of Jesus in the Jordan. Archbishop Fulton Sheen placed this unborn-meets-Unborn event in perspective, when he observed: "A Pentecost came before Pentecost."[4] The famous "leap" of unborn John foreshadows the responsiveness of the early Church members to the Holy Spirit when they spoke "in other tongues, as the Spirit gave them utterance" that first Pentecost day (Acts 2:4). As an unborn baby, John resorts to 'sign language' as "the Spirit gave (him) utterance". Father Fillion notes that John's leap:

> .....is not one of those natural movements sometimes occurring during pregnancy, but a supernatural and conscious movement,

> resulting from the joy which the future precursor, suddenly gifted with reason, experienced.....many Fathers and theologians have quite legitimately concluded that this privilege was then conferred on John the Baptist. Since her infant "leaped with joy", it must be that he was aware of what he was doing.......There is, however, a difference of opinion as to the duration of this favor, which, according to many authors, was merely transitory.[5]

John is "gifted with reason". God alone knows all that went through the mind of John at that turning point of his life. But we can also speculate as to whether John was being "gifted with faith" at that moment; giving new meaning to the expression, "a leap of faith". As to the possibility of being exceptionally gifted with reason, this is quite possible, for heaven's gifts are not always completely comprehensible to mortal man. And in relation to the virtue of faith, the faith assent similarly need not be seen as adult or mature or sophisticated. Indeed, did not Jesus teach that our faith should be simple and childlike, and that faith the size of a mustard seed would suffice? Jesus did not specify what childlike age He had in mind when He gave this teaching.

As Martin Luther points out: "To hold that a child believes, as St. John is an example, is not contrary to scripture."[6] Indeed the Gospel of Luke recounts that one day Jesus; "...rejoiced in the Holy Spirit and said, 'I thank thee, Father, Lord of heaven and earth, that thou hast hidden these things from the wise and understanding and revealed them to babes; yea, Father, for such was thy gracious will.'" (Lk 10:21). So, if some are reluctant to think of God as "imposing" Himself upon a tiny unborn baby, they may consider that, in fact, it wasn't an imposition at all but rather a beautiful blessing that even a baby could enjoy: an introduction to God's Grace and plan for the infant's life.

In this encounter God uses an unborn baby to proclaim the good news and further His Kingdom. Since Mary had kept her secret to herself, the unborn John is the first human being to bear witness to the Messiah! Why did God choose an unborn baby? Indeed, and why not? No physical human eyes – whether adult's or child's – could have seen the one-week-old Unborn Jesus. But the spiritual eyes of John saw, and then his not-so-spiritual leg(s) let fly a kick, which his mother politely calls a leap for joy. "Thou dost show me the path of life; in Thy presence there is fullness of joy "(Ps 16:11).

Recall that for about six months Elizabeth's home had been rather quiet: two elderly contemplatives, one unable to speak and the other in hiding from neighbor and kin (Lk 1:24). (Admittedly, their home may have also housed extended family members as was common in those days. In that case, it may not have been unusually quiet, but simply more subdued than normal.) The primary method Zechariah employed to communicate with Elizabeth was sign language. So likewise the unborn John invents a sign language of his own – and it works beautifully!

As God's last prophet in Israel prior to the coming of the Messiah, John's life would always be out of the ordinary. Moreover, he would grow in grace so that, responsive to the inspiration of the Holy Spirit, he would faithfully prepare the way of the Lord. And his prophetic office begins here and now in his mother's womb. This encounter prefigures the one to come thirty years later. Here Jesus fills John with the Holy Spirit within the life-giving intrauterine waters; three decades later Jesus will be baptized by John in the waters of the Jordan River. Here the Holy Spirit descends upon John in a baptism-like encounter; thirty years hence the Holy Spirit will descend upon Jesus as He comes up out of the baptismal waters. Following their baptismal experiences both are led by the Spirit into the wilderness (Lk 1:80, Mt 4:1).

We find in this encounter between the two unborn babies the answer to a question which would be asked of Jesus thirty years later by John himself: "Then Jesus came from Galilee to the Jordan to John, to be baptized by him. John would have prevented Him, saying, 'I need to be baptized by you, and do you come to me?' But Jesus answered him, 'Let it be so now; for thus it is fitting for us to fulfill all righteousness'"(Mt 3:13-15). One reason Jesus did not baptize John in the Jordan River was because He had already "baptized" him with the Holy Spirit, thirty years earlier while John was yet an unborn baby. So this unique encounter between them – while in their mothers' wombs – depicts the first time Jesus ever performed a baptism-like act upon anyone, and in a way it was this "baptism" of the Holy Spirit which John received that was the source and authentication for the baptisms he would administer three decades later. And also, as alluded to previously, this "baptism-like" experience of unborn John suggests the urgency of the Incarnation mission. Perhaps, further, it suggests the urgency of the Church's mission to baptize newborn infants soon after birth so that the Holy Spirit might be within their innocent hearts from the earliest possible moment and their futures consecrated and claimed for the Lord Jesus Christ (See endnote3; infant baptism). While John did not invite the Holy Spirit into his life, the Spirit entered him anyway, as a gratuitous gift from God.

From the first encounter to the second, three decades later, we witness how the fruit of joy – Messianic joy – characterizes the ever-unfolding plan of salvation. For when John was told that the people were now going to Jesus (actually to the disciples of Jesus) to be baptized, instead of to John (and his disciples), John exclaims: "He who has the bride is the bridegroom; the friend of the bridegroom, who stands and hears him, rejoices greatly at the bridegroom's voice; therefore this joy of mine is now full. He must increase, but I must decrease" (Jn 3:29-30).[7]

4. Elizabeth Is Filled with the Holy Spirit

Humble Elizabeth has an important role in this encounter; Fulton Sheen spoke of it in this way: "One of the most beautiful moments in history was that when pregnancy met pregnancy – when child bearers became the first heralds of the King of Kings."[8] God moves in mysterious ways. Fittingly, the elder of the two women present takes the lead in describing the great work God was doing in their midst. Most spiritual writers have held that Mary understood that it was not her mystery to reveal, but one God would make known. Thus the need for discretion made it unfitting for Mary to proclaim her secret to Elizabeth. However, Mother Angelica notes that "Like all fathers, God could not keep the wonderful secret too long. He had to tell someone, and that someone was Elizabeth. . . ."[9]

Elizabeth seems to have been awestruck by the immediate revelation she received at this moment. Some people would be similarly overwhelmed should a famous celebrity or world leader walk in their front door, but for Elizabeth there could have been nothing more momentous than the pregnant mother of the Messiah – carrying Him within her – entering her home. The Holy Spirit imparts to Elizabeth the gifts of knowledge and understanding, and she, who is full of good will and faith, is enlightened as to the meaning of what is occurring (Lk 1:42).

Archbishop Goodier notes that "... throughout His life the one desire of Jesus was that He should be discovered; that He should be discovered, and recognized, owned. For every step made in that discovery He was grateful; no man made it but met with reward overflowing. The one thread of interest running through the whole drama of His life is the growth of this discovery."[10] Unborn John and his mother Elizabeth share in this first discovery together, as if to remind us all that the first place Jesus should be discovered is in the family.

The words of testimony which Elizabeth spoke remind us of the famous statement of faith made by St. Peter many years later "You are the Christ, the Son of the living God.' And Jesus answered him, 'Blessed are you, Simon Bar-Jona! For flesh and blood has not revealed this to you, but my Father who is in heaven." (Mt 16:15-17) Flesh and blood did not reveal this astonishing mystery to Elizabeth either, rather the Father in heaven. Consider the astounding words of Elizabeth which introduce, for the first time, two titles: the title "Lord" to describe unborn baby Jesus, and the title "Mother of (the) Lord" to describe Mary.

But how did God unfold this mystery to Elizabeth? On the human level, we should remember that Zechariah had told her of John's vocation as precursor of the Messiah. She had been reflecting on the coming Messiah. Finally, having been "filled with the Holy Spirit" (Lk 1:42), Elizabeth's insight and words were a work of God. She was God's faithful instrument.

5. Elizabeth Greets Mary and Recounts John's Joy

The Bible prefaces Elizabeth's words with this introduction; ". . . .and she exclaimed with a loud cry. . . ." Wasn't Elizabeth elderly? Hadn't her recent life been somewhat subdued? Why then, "a loud cry"? Archbishop Sheen's description of the event as prefiguring Pentecost, would lead one to expect this encounter to be like Pentecost: vibrant, lively, and filled with enthusiasm and joy. How ironic that a meeting of two pregnant women and two unborn babies should be so forceful and unpredictable.

Elizabeth's greeting is humble, but not low key, for she cries out: "Blessed are you among women, and blessed is the fruit of your womb," thus assigning two blessings to Mary. A third blessing follows:

"And blessed is she who believed that there would be a fulfillment of what was spoken to her from the Lord."

The three blessings are all different, yet all related to Mary's extraordinary vocation as Mother of God. The first is similar to Gabriel's greeting in that it states a simple fact.

"Hail, full of grace, the Lord is with you!" (Gabriel)

"Blessed are you among women..." (Elizabeth)

Or, expressed in another way; "You are most blessed of all women." Elizabeth identifies Mary as the one woman in all of human history chosen by God for this most remarkable service to Israel and the entire world. She is mother to the Messiah. Even more, she is mother to the Lord. Never before had a mystery like this existed or been imagined. Elizabeth could see that God had exalted this maiden in an incomparable and incomprehensible way.

The second remarkable blessing follows upon the first quite naturally. Mary carries within her the Lord. What more can be said? "And why is this granted me, that the mother of my Lord should come to me?" These comments of Elizabeth reveal a shifting focus, from Mary to Unborn Jesus, back to Mary then back to the Lord. Here writer Charles Hoffman portrays a prophetic breakthrough: "Now Elizabeth didn't recognize what was in Mary's womb as a 'fetus.' No One less than God the Holy Spirit gave Elizabeth the gift to recognize that what was alive in her cousin's womb, was already a person. And that person was her Lord (God)."[11] Elizabeth – pregnant and inspired – proclaims the Personhood of the Son of God and her allegiance to Him with the words "my Lord". The Lord is present, not potentially but here and now!

Elizabeth is keenly aware of her unworthiness to witness these holy mysteries of Almighty God. She feels out of place. Her husband Zechariah had been contacted by God's own archangel but had responded poorly when asked to participate in the Messianic plan. Neither had Elizabeth realized how holy and pleasing to God her young kinswoman was, and for this lack of perception, too, she may have felt some sense of failure. Why would God bring His deepest secret, His greatest act into her home, and why was God's Mercy directed towards her, Elizabeth? All of this was beyond her wildest imaginings and completely unfathomable.

The third blessing unveils Mary's greatest quality: "And blessed is she who believed" (Lk 1:45). The Holy Spirit wanted Mary's belief from the moment of Gabriel's revelation to be known. She had not doubted, as Zechariah and probably all of us would have. She didn't hesitate as many of us do in the smallest of our undertakings. She forthrightly – we could say matter-of-factly – believed!

The first and third sentences spoken by Elizabeth address Mary as "you". The second sentence is almost like a heavenward prayer of inquiry: "And why is this granted me.....?" But the fourth and final sentence uttered by Elizabeth stands alone: neither addressed to Mary as you, nor to heaven as a prayer. This prophetic testimony is to benefit future believers. Elizabeth exclaims; "And blessed is she who believed.....what was spoken to her from the Lord."

These words indicate that Mary believed the message she received from Gabriel: once overshadowed by the Spirit she believed her holy child to be the Son of God. During the following days, though she had no one to confide in or to go to for advice, she continued to believe! She was an improbable choice – yet she believed! The way by which she conceived was unprecedented, and there was no physical sign of her pregnancy – yet she believed! She was young and of very humble origins – yet she believed! Her betrothed was a simple carpenter of no consequence – yet she believed! Mary trusted God with all her heart, all her mind, all her soul, and all her strength.

6. Mary Responds to This Greeting

> And Mary said,
> "My soul magnifies the Lord,
> and my spirit rejoices in God my Savior,
> for he has regarded the low estate of his handmaiden.
> For behold, henceforth all generations
> will call me blessed... Luke 1:46-48

Mary's spontaneous response has been the subject of countless words of commentary over the past two thousand years. So the observations here will be limited in scope, focusing on her perspective as the pregnant mother of the Lord. Pope John Paul II spoke of her response in this way: "Adoration of God full of joy, and joy full of adoration of God: this is the state of her blessed soul, these are the deepest sentiments that feed her heart....There appears in the Magnificat that gratitude full of humility which is an infallible sign of the encounter with the living God." [12]

The opening line is striking; "My soul magnifies the Lord...." She is perhaps conscious of the transparent joy radiating from within her heart and womb. She cannot hide her joy, so she simply allows it to reflect to those who would receive it; as the soft moonlight might glisten and dance upon the surface of a lake so the glory of her God is magnified by her still and peaceful soul. Hers is a childlike soul, all the better to magnify her unborn baby Lord. But she doesn't say possessively "my Lord": rather she sets Him apart for all to behold saying "the Lord", and so confirms Elizabeth's testimony to her son's identity.

Mary's song received its Latin name, the Magnificat, from the opening line. Christians throughout the ages have wrestled with the mystery of Mary's motherhood and its impact upon her life. How does Mary's soul "magnify" the Lord? Cardinal Berulle unfolds this singular relationship for us:

> She bears the impression of and a share in his divine actions. She exists not through her own light and love, but through the light, love and activity of Jesus who draws her into union with himself. He also draws her out of herself and her own interior actions so that she might live in him and be the bearer of his holy activities through a sort of gentle, exalted and powerful impression by which the Mother is enraptured by her Son, the Virgin by Jesus. Thus Jesus is living in the Virgin and hers is the first soul in which he established his life. The Virgin's proper role is to be attentive to the interior and spiritual life of her Son and to be a pure capacity for Jesus, filled with Jesus.[13]

The poet Gerard Manley Hopkins hints at the reality of this mystery:

> All things rising, all things sizing
> Mary sees, sympathizing
> With that world of good
> Nature's motherhood.
>
> Their magnifying of each its kind
> With delight calls to mind
> How she did in her stored
> Magnify the Lord.

This ecstasy all through mothering earth
Tells Mary her mirth till Christ's birth
To remember and exultation
In God who was her salvation.[14]

Mary's relationship to her baby, and His influence upon her life is one of the most beautiful mysteries of God's infancy. From the words of Gabriel, Elizabeth, and most significantly Mary herself, we see that she was filled with the Holy Spirit, exuded the joy of the Spirit, and was the living example – rather the prototype – of that ancient proverb: "A glad heart makes a cheerful countenance" (Prov 15:13).

Not only her soul, but also her countenance magnified the Lord within her. Those open to the working of the Spirit of God within their lives are generally also known for their openness to life and other people. This outlook would be consistent with what we know about Mary (who, we must remember, had "found favor with God" [Lk 1:30]), and also with what appears to have been her manner throughout some rather tumultuous events: the journey to Bethlehem when more than eight months pregnant, giving birth in primitive conditions, the warnings of danger and lengthy sojourn in the foreign land of Egypt, and finally the return accompanied by an additional warning regarding where to dwell, and so on. A hallmark of this openness to God, to life, and to people is that healthy naturalness in one's behavior that is free and genuine.

Perhaps a contrast between Mary and Moses might help us in gaining perspective. Recall that after being alone with God on Mount Sinai for forty days, the face of Moses the lawgiver shone and it made the people afraid (Ex 34:29-30). In the case of Mary – who had been virtually and most intimately alone with God for perhaps a week – the effect of this proximity is exactly the opposite. As Mercy-bearer (rather than Law-giver), her manner is all gentleness, making people hopeful rather than fearful. When she greeted Elizabeth, in some blessed way, her voice "magnified" His voice, as if to foreshadow what her Son would explain to future disciples: "He who hears you hears me" (Lk 10:16).

Mary's Magnificat refers again to herself; "for He has regarded the low estate of His handmaiden..." Her comment here is most telling. She had previously identified herself to Gabriel as "the handmaid of the

Lord" and now she is careful to once again use this term to explain her role to her cousin. But now she has further personalized her role of service for she refers to herself here as handmaiden to "God my Savior".

Gabriel twice referred to the Father of Jesus as "the Most High" and now, in juxtaposition, Mary makes clear that she is "most lowly" (Lk 1:48). But what can bridge this infinite distance between God and humanity? Mercy! God's Mercy Incarnate!

The central theme of Mary's Magnificat is God's mercy.[15] She explicitly proclaims: "And His mercy is on those who fear him....He has helped his servant Israel, in remembrance of his mercy" (Lk 1:50, 54). Here in the Magnificat (and again in Zechariah's song, Lk 1:68-79) the theme of God's mercy is so prevalent in conjunction with the Incarnation that mercy may be identified as another incarnational virtue. In chapter one, we spoke of humility and obedience as specifically incarnational virtues exemplified by Unborn Jesus as He came into the world. Here is another corresponding virtue.

Perhaps one last observation is in order regarding Mary's song. Many have failed to appreciate the Magnificat's message, perhaps because some verses and references may seem foreign or confusing, if not downright unmerciful: "...He has scattered the proud...He has put down the mighty from their thrones...the rich He has sent empty away"(Lk 1:51-53). There is the element of warning in these references, and as any parent will tell you, most warnings are given out of love and concern. The Magnificat seems to recapitulate all of human history. While Mary recounts the promises God made to Abraham and his posterity "for ever"; she acknowledges the mercy of God "from generation to generation", and in relation to her Son, she knows that "all generations" will call her blessed. She sees the futile human perspective of history as one government follows another, symbolized by "the mighty" and their "thrones", in contrast to the Messiah, Prince of Peace, whose Kingdom is everlasting. She points to the emptiness of "the rich" in contrast to the Creator of all things and Lord of all. Indeed, there is an attempt here to correct those abiding human misconceptions about history by shifting our focus to "He who is mighty" (and has "strength with His arm") and away from "the proud" who might think themselves "the mighty".

At the conclusion of the Magnificat, the listener is left with the distinct impression that the great strength of the Almighty lies hidden both within Mary and in His never ending mercy. And so we can see that Mary's song, inspired by the Holy Spirit, and especially suited for the lips of Mary, is not boastful or superficial poetry, but a timeless message from within Mary to a waiting needy world, a preview then and a reminder now, of the message Christ came to preach; "Repent, for the kingdom of heaven is at hand" (Mt 4:17).

A New Creation

If one viewed the actions of this scene from a distance, without hearing any of the words being spoken, the occurrence would be mundane, perhaps quaint, but of little interest. But in this mystical encounter the Spirit enlightens minds, anticipates words, and anoints those involved with supernatural gifts. God acts and people respond. And the people also act in unison with the Spirit, so that they participate in fulfilling God's Holy designs.

Thus this warm reunion of kinsfolk becomes much more. Within the womb of the younger woman is the New Adam, bringing a New Covenant and establishing a New Creation. Within the womb of the elder woman is the witness who will bear testimony to these realities. The elder represents the long waiting for the fulfillment of the promise. The handmaiden carries within heart and womb the seed of a holy new order. We are reminded here of Eden, its destiny and innocence lost, because here is its renewal, not as yet a rebirth, but conceived and exuberantly expected.

Two inspired women, two active unborn male babies, two sexes, two generations, two families visited by God's Archangel, two miraculous pregnancies, two quiet men offstage, and two levels of activity, the spiritual and the physical: these recall an instance when a "second creation" had been planned. Within the Ark of Noah all manner of creatures paired, male and female, two by two, preserved within its dark safety, under a deluge from Heaven prefiguring baptism (Gen 6:7-9.20 and I Pet 3:20-21).[16] Now within ark-like wombs we see the promise of the true New Creation.

This scene reminds us that every pregnancy is a gift of new life from God. Every unborn baby is new innocence shaped by nature's hand and then given to humankind with the challenge and responsibility of preserving and protecting the inherent goodness of each child.

This scene of hopefulness ushers in the Incarnation Mission of God's Son with praise and prophecy, with gentleness and loving embrace. The welcome extended here to the Unborn Son of God is a sign of the recognition and welcome which should be afforded Him everywhere and at all times, in every unborn child.

CHAPTER THREE ENDNOTES

1 God acts first. See I Jn 4:19 and Rom 5:8.

2 Rev. Frederick W. Faber, C. Orat., D.D., *The Blessed Sacrament* (Baltimore, MD: John Murphy Company, circa 1855), 162-163.

3 Infant baptism has been a consistent practice since Apostolic times. In the writings of the early Church Fathers there are numerous references to this common practice. Martin Luther passionately defended the practice in a34-page treatise he wrote in 1528 entitled *Concerning Rebaptism*; LW, Vol.40, translated by Conrad Bergendoff. Luther lists numerous arguments in favor of infant baptism in this unique document. In1758 John Wesley published *A Preservative Against Unsettled Notions in Religion*, which contained an extensive defense of the practice of infant baptism. In fact, Wesley says infants "have a right to baptism" and that it is "our bounden duty" to baptize our children. Albert Coutler, editor, *John Wesley* (New York: Oxford University Press, 1964), 317-332. In a more modern discussion, Presbyterian Francis A. Schaeffer defended the age-old practice of infant baptism admonishing parents: "Take advantage of this God-given privilege of infant baptism." [F. Schaeffer, *Baptism*, (Lawrenceville,GA: Christian Education and Publications, 2004), 15.

4 Archbishop Fulton Sheen, Ph.D., D.D., *The World's First Love* (Garden City, NY: Doubleday & Company, Inc., 1956), 31.

5 Rev. L.C. Fillion, S.S., *The Life Of Christ*, trans. Rev. Newton Thompson, S.T.D. (St. Louis, MO: B. Herder Book Co., 1940), 268-269.

6 Martin Luther, *Concerning Rebaptism*, LW, Vol. 40, trans. Conrad Bergendoff (Philadelphia, PA: Muhlenberg Press, 1962), 242.

7 Jesus is the bridegroom, and the bride is represented by the people of Israel going to Him for baptism, and John is the friend of the bridegroom. Shortly afterwards John would be arrested for criticizing a false "bridegroom" and the false bride he had taken; namely, Herod and Herodias (Mt 14:3-4). As Jesus would die for His bride, so John died for criticizing Herod's.

8 Archbishop Fulton Sheen, Ph.D., D.D., *The World's First Love*, op. cit., p.29.

9 Mother M. Angelica, O.S.C., *The Promised Woman* (Birmingham, AL: Journey Into Scripture, Catholic Family Missionary Alliance, Our Lady of Angels Monastery, 1978), 15.

10 Archbishop Alban Goodier, S.J., *The Public Life of Our Lord Jesus Christ*, Vol. One (New York: P.J. Kennedy & Sons, 1944), 244.

11 Charles Hoffman, *The Holy Rosary Rich in Jewish Tradition* (Santa Barbara, CA: Queenship Publishing Company, 1998), 4.

12 Pope John Paul II, Angelus Message, Dec16, 1984.

13 William M. Thompson, ed., *Berulle And The French School, Selected Writings,* trans. Lowell M. Glendon, S.S. (Mahwah, NJ: Paulist Press, 1989), 169.

14 Rev. Gerard Manley Hopkins, S.J., *The May Magnificat.*

15 Mary's Magnificat has been compared with Hannah's Song (I Sam 2:1-10). There are similarities in language, and both songs belong to the same genre. Both women have special sons who are offered to God's service. But while Hannah's song of justice and judgment is an Old Covenant song, Mary's is a New Covenant song telling God's mercy. The tone of the former is satisfaction in God's execution of His might and justice, while the tone of the latter is joyful and hopes in the promises of God.

16 What might be referred to as "creation terminology" is repeatedly used in the account about Noah; cf. Gen 7:4,10,11, 8:13,17, 9:1-3,7-10,19-20.

4

The Visitation: A Three-Month Retreat

And Mary remained with her about three months...
Luke 1:56

When Mary arrives at the home of Elizabeth and Zechariah, the Unborn Son of God is probably about a week old. As we have considered already, the action begins immediately – within seconds of her arrival – and it is initiated by the unborn Messiah and responded to by the unborn prophet in unison with the Holy Spirit. The tone established for this ninety-day visit, as we have already discussed, might simply be stated as joy. Joy in the fulfillment of God's promises! Messianic Joy!

The focus of the ninety-day visit was preparation. God had called all of these individuals to serve Him in a most extraordinary manner, and before proceeding further God prepared them for the months and years ahead. Elizabeth and Zechariah were well disposed, after six quiet months spent in large measure listening, praying and reflecting. Mary was young and eager to continue as the Lord willed. But all three needed this special time with the Word Incarnate. And paradoxically, unborn John would now be prepared by the unborn Lord to years later return the favor and "prepare the way of the Lord" (Is 40:3).

"and a little child shall lead them" (Is 11:6)

We can not say definitively what Unborn Jesus did while still in the womb of His mother. But we can ponder these events with faith and love. What was this Divine Presence like within Mary's womb, nestled under the beacon of her heart? "The flame of fire in the burning bush was a figure of Jesus in Mary's sacred womb.... So He still speaks as if concealed in Mary's womb...".[1]

Truly, this personal human presence of the Son of God within the womb of Mary was sacred and powerful, while also subtle and gentle. In speaking of the two natures in the single person of Jesus Christ in the mystery of the Incarnation, St. Fulgence of Ruspe (467-527 A.D.) observed: "Nevertheless, the divinity did not consume the humanity, nor did the humanity change the divinity into something else...".[2] This comment recalls the burning bush, engulfed in fire that "did not consume" the bush (Ex 3:2-3). So, "the divinity did not consume the humanity" in the person of Jesus, nor did the divinity of the child consume the humanity of the mother. Perhaps the difference between the bush ablaze and the mother expectant is that the former is a spectacular miracle, whereas the latter is mystifyingly tender and meek. Moses was frightened by the spectacle (Ex 3:6), but who could be frightened of this young and thoughtful handmaid, Mary? She did not obscure the presence of the Son of God within her by arrogance, vanity, or any peculiar personal characteristics. Her naturally simple human ways were ideally matched with these supernatural divine ways of God's providence.

Perhaps a final analogy might help us to further appreciate the power of this Unborn presence. Consider how the fire in a fireplace within a small cabin draws all who enter towards its glowing warmth. In a similar spiritual sense, the Unborn Son of God would have attracted His hosts – Elizabeth and Zechariah – to Himself. For their part, remaining humble and receptive, they would sense the tranquility of His Being and their open hearts would be enflamed by His nearness. Similarly, recall how the woman who touched the hem of His garment, while a crowd bustled about Him, was instantly healed by the Power in Him. Crowds were attracted to Him. For those of good will, His presence was attractiveness itself, and no doubt His physical presence would have become the new focal point of this small home.

The Formative Development of Unborn Jesus

Mary's visit coincides roughly with the first trimester of her pregnancy. Truly the first trimester of every baby's life should be singled out as the most remarkable three months of a lifetime. For Jesus, as it is for every human being, the period included extremely rapid and complex physiological development.

The growth rate, relatively speaking, was frantic. The first distinctive parts of His Body to be formed would have been the heart and head. At three weeks they were primitively functional, but by six weeks their form is clearly distinctive. Pope Pius XII has stated that from the moment of Our Lord's conception. "Immediately the Heart of Jesus, ever to be adored, has begun to pulsate with love, divine and human."[3] The Love of God Incarnate did not wait for a physical human organ to join its urgent surging beat for love of us! But certainly once the physical human organ was in place it too, in perfect unison, took up this pulse of eternal love.

By eight weeks His unborn body was fully defined in its formation, although still extremely tiny in size. By the end of the third month His other organs would have also been functioning. Weighing merely an ounce, His Body was delicately formed and complete – just a spiritual stone's throw from Golgotha, where one day He would offer this body as a sacrifice.

Physically the unborn Jesus was like other unborn infants throughout this first trimester, but in spiritual capacities, Pius XII again reminds us, He was singular: ". . . .the Body of Jesus Christ, formed by the work of the Holy Spirit in the womb of the Virgin Mary, enjoyed in the fullest degree the power of feeling and perceiving, more perfectly in fact than the bodies of all other men." [4] This is an interesting observation even though it is extremely difficult to measure, by degrees, a person's feelings or perceptions, and even more difficult still – if not completely impossible – to measure these capacities in unborn infants. Nonetheless, we acknowledge two points here 1. that we are considering a very profound mystery, and 2. that Jesus possessed a capacity for feeling and perceiving above what is normally found in humans – particularly other unborn humans.

> He is God and therefore there can be nothing imperfect about Him; from the first moment of the Word being made flesh in the womb of His Mother till "she brought forth her first-born Son" on Christmas day, His faculties, His reason, His intelligence, His sensibilities were all in a state of perfection; He knew the past, the present, and the future; and He, the Source of grace, was pouring forth

> grace on all around Him. Directly we understand this, we feel that we must draw near, not only to adore but to sympathize, to wonder, to love, to learn, to imitate. For those who understand the Incarnation, His work did not begin on Christmas Day, but on the Feast of the Annunciation....[5]

Perhaps to linger on the perfections of Unborn Jesus for a moment would be helpful. In His adult life, He was able to love people more than anyone else could hope to and to teach better than any other teacher ever would. Also, He saw better than all others the goodness and potential (as well as the sins and weaknesses) of those people with whom He came in contact. So too, one may attribute similar capabilities to Him at His earlier ages (and at least in comparison to others of those same ages) whether as an adolescent, a little boy, a newborn baby or an unborn baby.

Like all unborn babies in the womb, Jesus was physically active in a secret way, but unlike other unborn babies, He was spiritually active: His redemptive activity had already begun. The tiny, young Unborn Jesus had accepted the normal limitations found by infants in the womb and made those same constraints His own. He, however, did not stop loving with a divine love because He was Incarnate – to have done so would have contradicted His divine nature, and defied the very purpose of the Incarnation. St. Peter Julian Eymard wrote that: "This love inflamed His Heart from the first moment of His conception until His last breath and, since His resurrection, has not ceased nor will ever cease doing so."[6]

The Heart of Jesus has been the object of a lively devotion within the Catholic tradition for many centuries. Scholars have traced it back to the early years of the Church: perhaps it originated in the beautiful and intimate invitation Jesus offered when He said: "Come to me, all who labor and are heavy laden, and I will give you rest. Take my yoke upon you, and learn from me; *for I am gentle and lowly in heart, and you will find rest for your souls.* For my yoke is easy, and my burden is light" (Emphasis added) (Mt 11:28-30).

He offers rest, not just physical or mental rest, but a complete spiritual rest for our very souls. Where? How? By turning our whole attention to His Heart. There we can obtain a spiritual education – "learn from me" – simply by resting upon that ever gentle and lowly heart and listening as St. John did at the Last Supper (Jn 13:23). "It is important that in our veneration we should not separate the Heart of Jesus from the divinity of the Man-God.....and the worship we pay to the Heart has not its final end in that Heart, but in the adorable Person Who possesses it and Who has united it to Himself forever.....for when we honor His Heart, we mean to praise all the actions and the whole life of Jesus Christ, which are but an outpouring of His Heart."[7]

And so we picture the unborn baby Jesus within His mother's womb, skin almost transparent in these early weeks of human life, and His Heart, not yet hidden by a thicker, more developed skin, but visible, actually throbbing, pulsing with divine love for us! This is the miniature reservoir of that one commodity that could purchase the salvation of the entire human race, the blood of God Himself! This Precious Blood is separate and different from His mother's. A small delicate vial of heavenly medicine. It is a tiny Heart, but proportionately – compared to the rest of its body, during the first and second months – it measures up to nine times the size of the adult heart. Appropriately, the Heart of Unborn Jesus (and His head) dominated His Body: for the Incarnation is about God's Love for us.

The contents of this little vial – the blood of Christ – was the ink with which the New Covenant would be written. It was being produced within the tiny Heart of Unborn Jesus and it was flowing like new wine within His compact body, already beginning to age for that day of its final outpouring. Years later the early church would hold Christ's blood in the highest reverence and speak with awe of its effects (see Paul's comments for example: Eph 1:7,2:13, Col 1:20). Today Christians boldly acknowledge that Christ's blood is the currency which purchased their ransom (I Pet 1:18-19), and humbly make childlike claim upon His Precious Blood for their everlasting salvation. Likewise, Christians can follow the stream of His blood back to its source, to its point of origin (physiologically and chronologically) and also lay claim to the very Heart of Jesus Christ and "his steadfast love (which) endures for ever" (Ps 100:5).

Not only was the Heart of Unborn Jesus proportionally large in physical size, but – like that of all unborn infants – it beat at a much faster rate than the adult heart (roughly twice as fast) as if to leave no doubt as to its quickening desires and designs towards the human family.[8] As the Child, quickened with life, stirred within His mother's womb, so the Heart of the Child quickened by the Spirit, stirred within the Child's Body.

Now if the adult Heart of Jesus was gentle and lowly (Mt 11), how much more so the tiny, developing baby Heart of Jesus? Lowly in size and shape, gentle as a baby's alone could be. But if humanly frail, by no means limited. Think of how St. Paul explains one of the mysterious qualities of the Spirit: "Likewise the Spirit helps us in our weakness; for we do not know how to pray as we ought, but the Spirit himself intercedes for us with sighs too deep for words." (Rom 8:26) And are babies not capable of "sighs too deep for words"? And the Unborn Baby Jesus? Paul's next sentence explains still a little bit more: "...and he who searches the hearts of men knows what is the mind of the Spirit..."

In other words, God the Father and God the Holy Spirit communicate without the use of human words, which are limited in their capacity to communicate. Unborn Jesus likewise communicates in a divine manner we will never comprehend in this lifetime. We should not limit the power of God by misapplying modest human perceptions to its analysis. For as St. Ambrose (born c. 334, died 397 A.D.) observed concerning Mary and her unborn Child: "Her Son, who is beyond our understanding, is active in His mother in a way beyond our understanding."[9]

Unborn John Encounters the Unborn Lord

John benefited spiritually from the presence of Unborn Jesus directly and also indirectly. The most striking direct benefit was described in the last chapter: the reception of the Holy Spirit which made John physically leap for joy.

But throughout the three months, the continual presence of the Unborn Lord a mere breath or heartbeat away reaffirmed the effect of his "baptism-like" experience on John's soul. In some spiritual way, beyond our ability to fathom, the intensity of its impact was prolonged as its full significance was eternally imprinted upon the various faculties of his soul. The fire of the Holy Spirit enflamed his intellect, seared his conscience, enkindled his memory, and ignited his will. John was a prophet destined to die a martyr's death for speaking out as the same Spirit would later give him utterance.

His "contact" with, or physical proximity to, Unborn Jesus was a function of his mother's relationship with the Lord's mother. As the two mothers drew close to talk or pray together, might not the grace of the Lord have been like a quiet, whispering wind breezing across John's soul?

Indirectly, the lasting effects of the numerous blessings received by his parents during this visit would also be conveyed to him over time by their instruction and influence. An example of this shows up in his adult years as we note the tremendous deference and respect he showed to Jesus on a number of occasions.

Elizabeth Is Strengthened for Her New Role

At an elderly age, Elizabeth embarked on the path of motherhood. In seclusion for six months, probably her only companion was her mute husband Zechariah, who – we might suspect – was himself not in the most serene frame of mind. It had been a strange and lonely six months: perhaps the most difficult months of her life. A bittersweet time. Her husband was still distressed at having doubted Gabriel: as his wife, she was yoked to his troubled thoughts and sad countenance. With whom could she share her joy? To whom could she vent her anxieties about her son's childhood, and from whom could she receive encouraging words in return? Who could understand her situation and nurture hope in her new mother's heart? And who could lift the spirits of her husband? Enter Mary: her young faithful heart near exploding with the Holy Spirit and the exuberant joy of miraculous motherhood and intimate knowledge of the Messianic mission. Mary's companionship and support were a great blessing for Elizabeth.

But more important than Mary, the Lord arrives with His divine companionship. Now Elizabeth could pour out her heart.....and then listen with a renewed heart as the Word spoke to her. Conversations had been banished from her house and silence had been a constant companion, but now the very Word of God Himself came in through the front door and dwelt in the center of her home.

Zechariah: Restored in the Presence of God

The priest Zechariah had been the first person told of the Messiah's impending mission to the House of Israel. That God willed this is understandable as he was a faithful and holy priest. Zechariah represents the remnant of faithful souls within Israel awaiting the Messiah. The reader is encouraged to read and ponder the sobering account of the Archangel Gabriel's appearance to Zechariah (Lk 1:8-23).

Gabriel's initial greeting had been full of tenderness as he recounted God's attentiveness to the prayers of both Zechariah and Elizabeth. He then proclaimed the conception and future mission of Zechariah's son John. As the Archangel details the tremendous prophetic office to be held by John we are in awe of the spectacular manner in which God is delivering this most solemn message to this chosen priest as he devoutly ministers at the altar in the temple.

But Zechariah confronts the Archangel with a doubting question: "How shall I know this? For I am an old man, and my wife is advanced in years." Suddenly, this joyous breathtaking event sours. Zechariah had fallen prey to the common temptation of intellectualizing the movements and blessings of God in one's life. Instead of responding with faith and trust, Zechariah skeptically questioned the Will of God. Human impertinence is the ever-present temptation for all who are "well educated".

The Archangel has no choice but to put aside the rest of the message as it was intended to be delivered. He delivers instead a brief angelic rebuke: "*I am Gabriel, who stand in the presence of God and I was sent to speak to you, and to bring you this good news.*" (Emphasis added) If an angel can scowl this one must have. Gabriel does not even acknowledge, let alone answer, Zechariah's question that was born of doubt.

The divine message has, in effect, been cut short and there is nothing left to say. Indeed, the Angel will see to it that Zechariah has nothing else to say for a very long time: ". . . . .you will be silent and unable to speak until the day that these things come to pass. . . ." And when would "these things come to pass"? Zechariah had no way of knowing when, exactly, he would regain his speech. Would it be in nine months, or nine years or even nineteen years? And even after Elizabeth was unquestionably pregnant, Zechariah could still not be sure of when he would speak again. Fillion's *Life of Christ* recounts the event in this way: "Why, then, is (Zechariah) treated so severely? It is because the angel, in showing that he read the priest's heart, since he knew the object of his interior prayer, was by that fact accredited as God's envoy.

He deserved to have his words taken; it is (Zechariah's) doubt, not his request that was punished."[10]

More should be expected of a holy priest, wise in years who had dedicated his life to serving God. Now he had failed God miserably while serving at the holy temple altar. So he returns from his temple service a broken man. He has failed God and his people; he sees himself a failure. He had even failed his wife, for together they had prayed for a child and now when God mercifully grants their prayer, Zechariah disbelieves. It seemed as if, in an instant he had brought himself to near spiritual ruin.

Five hundred years before, his namesake the prophet Zechariah – who was also a priest – had written at length about the coming of the Messiah. "Sing and rejoice, O daughter of Zion; for lo, I come and I will dwell in the midst of you, says the Lord" (Zech 2:1). Zechariah of Ain-Karim, would have had a keen interest in the prophecies and teaching concerning the long awaited Messiah, but now by his own doubt and lack of faith he had rebuffed the exalted Archangel Gabriel, the same angel who had appeared to the great prophet Daniel. For more than a thousand years Israel had been longing for this act of divine intervention. The inaugural message of this, the Messianic Age, was destined for the ears of one man only, and now that chosen man was covered by shame, in a state of shock and his spirit shattered! "O that today you would hearken to his voice! Harden not your hearts, as at Meribah, as on the day at Massah in the wilderness, when your fathers tested me, and put me to the proof, though they had seen my work" (Ps 95:7-9).

And so for the next six months, prior to the arrival of Mary (and Jesus), Zechariah was a man ashamed, begging God to forgive him for his stubborn and hardened heart. He was acutely aware of his sinfulness and weakness and would have prayed often, readily identifying with many of the Psalms. "O Lord, rebuke me not in thy anger, nor chasten me in thy wrath...! I am utterly bowed down and prostrate; all the day I go about mourning" (Ps 38:1,6). Poor Zechariah. He would not be the last believer to doubt, hinder or protest God's plan of salvation. "Against thee, thee only have I sinned, and done that which is evil in thy sight, so that thou art justified in thy sentence and blameless in thy judgment" (Ps 51:4). Prior to Mary's visit, his only companions were his loyal wife and his conscience. The silence was spiritually deafening – overwhelming. "For God alone my soul waits in silence; from Him comes my salvation...For God alone my soul waits in silence, for my hope is from Him" (Ps 62:1,5).

Finally, with Mary came hope. Literally, physically, supernaturally, prophetically. A great ray of light broke through the clouds of Zechariah's thoughts and musings. As he could witness God fulfilling His promises to Israel – in spite of his own obstinacy – hope began to grow in him and even the courage to believe more fiercely that yes, God could forgive him, God would forgive him and even rely on him again.

> So even to old age and gray hairs,
> O God, do not forsake me,
> till I proclaim thy might
> to all the generations to come....
> Thou who hast made me see many sore troubles
> wilt revive me again;
> from the depths of the earth
> thou wilt bring me up again.....
> I will sing praises to thee with the lyre,
> O Holy One of Israel.
> My lips will shout for joy,
> when I sing praises to thee;
> my soul also, which thou hast rescued. Ps 71:18-23

For Zechariah this visit was a wonderful gift from God, an indescribable consolation. And in three short months his lips would again sing aloud the praises of God his Savior.

Mary: Formed from Within by the One Forming Within Her

The Mission with which Mary had been entrusted was in every detail singular. God in His Wisdom wanted Mary to be uniquely prepared for her mission. Just as Jesus would later spend forty days alone in the wilderness at the outset of His public ministry, so too Mary now had ninety days of special preparation at the outset of her ministry as Mother to the Messiah.

Perhaps the prayer of Saint John Eudes might shed a little light on several aspects of this first preparatory trimester of faith.

> O Jesus, when I consider Thee in this mystery, I see by the light of faith that Thou dost entertain most exalted thoughts and great designs upon her in whom the Incarnation was accomplished, and that Thou dost indeed effect great and marvelous things in her. O Jesus, I adore Thy first thoughts, Thy first acts of love and movements of grace, of light and of eminent sanctity which Thou didst produce in Thy Blessed Mother at the moment of Thy Incarnation. So, too, do I adore the first acts of adoration, praise and love of the most admirable Mother for the Most Adorable Son. Blessed be Thou, O Jesus, Son of Mary, for all the wonders Thou didst work....[11]

Mary was being prepared by the One within her, Who, like a sculptor, was sculpting her from the inside, using invisible instruments: graces, blessings, gifts and fruits of the Spirit. Her heart, as well as her womb, was pregnant with hope. As she continued to mature in holiness, she became even more sensitive to God working within her. This prepared her to be sensitive to the Son of God in the future as He sat upon her lap, crawled on the floor, and in a thousand other ways.

The umbilical cord ensured the continual physical exchange between mother and Child. Food, oxygen and other substances pass from the mother to the Child through a single vein, and waste material passes from the Child to the mother through two arteries. Likewise there was a continual spiritual exchange between creature and Creator akin to that of the physical, but yet more profound. While mother nourished and sustained her Child on the physical level, the Child nourished and sustained His mother on the spiritual level. From her and within her, He was physically formed, but by Him and within Him she was being spiritually formed. Mary, like the rest of us, was dependent upon Almighty God: "In him we live and move and have our being...for we are indeed his offspring" (Act 17:28).

But with regards to Unborn Jesus, a slight paraphrase of the above reminds us that the reverse was true in the physical order: 'In her He lived and moved and had His being...for He was indeed her offspring."[12]

The relationship between Mary and Jesus is unparalleled, especially now during pregnancy. Yet, as Lutheran Professor David S. Yeago reveals, this uniqueness makes their relationship meaningful to all Christians:

> Mary's paradigmatic role is different in kind from that of her Son: she is not the Redeemer but the prototype of the redeemed; she is not the one in whom we participate but the paradigm of that par-

> ticipation. Jesus the Messiah in his dying and rising is alone the *forma formans*, the form-giving form, the one in whom all things hang together (Col 1:17) and around whose crucified and risen person the whole creation is to be blessedly configured. Mary by contrast is the *forma formata*, the form that has received formation, the prototype precisely of those who are not the Savior, but cling to him by faith, and on the way of faith's pilgrimage endure the protracted inscription of his image on their being.[13]

In these beautiful designs of Providence – wherein supernaturally Mary clings to her unborn Son and naturally He clings to her – we behold a twofold message reminding us of the lengths to which God has gone in the Incarnation to be with us and the lengths to which we should go in reciprocating.

Ministering to Each Other

For three months these five persons lived peaceably together. None of the three males spoke until after John's birth. The two women spoke freely and deeply, but not necessarily frequently. By way of writing tablet (Lk 2:63), probably a thin board covered with wax, Zechariah could have participated in their conversations. We assume that Zechariah could hear perfectly well and that his presence would not have hindered conversation between Elizabeth and Mary.[14]

Remembering that Zechariah was an elderly and holy priest, we can assume that he was well versed in the scriptures. Further, following his angelic encounter, Zechariah had ample opportunity and increasing motivation, during the ensuing six months – prior to Mary's visit – to further study the various Messianic texts in scripture and to meditate and pray over them. So when the mother of the Messiah appeared at his front door, Zechariah would probably be an expert on the topic. We can picture then, a certain intellectual attraction between the elderly Zechariah and the young mother, Mary. She, wanting to know more and more about all the scriptural references to her Son, and Zechariah – who had let God down before and now had a second chance to serve faithfully in the Messianic Mission – would be eager to share his knowledge and insights.

Mary was indeed already cognizant of the scriptural prophecies and descriptions of the Messiah. But Zechariah could have deepened her understanding of these things and also provided additional insight and perspective based on his priestly training and personal study. Of course, Zechariah also told Mary (or perhaps Elizabeth recounted) the details concerning his visit from Gabriel. (Likely Mary later relayed this information to Luke for inclusion in his Gospel.)

When we look at this tiny gathering we see, in the adults, examples of the faithful Israelites St. Paul writes of: "So too at the present time there is a remnant, chosen by grace" (Rom 11:5). Gabriel's visits indicate God's favor with these kinsfolk. Their way of life was exemplary before the Incarnation; afterwards it was crowned with grace from the Messiah within their midst. They were a prefigurement of the house churches to follow in the early centuries of Christianity. The diverse fruits of the Holy Spirit were manifested in their daily life together. The following counsel by St. Paul could have been derived by observing these three adults living in unity those three short months: "Let love be genuine; hate what is evil, hold fast to what is good; love one another with brotherly affection; outdo one another in showing honor. Never flag in zeal, be aglow with the Spirit, serve the Lord. Rejoice in your hope, be patient in tribulation, be constant in prayer" (Rom 12:9-12).

The spiritual writer, Ronda Chervin, has described the Visitation as "an icon of friendship:" ". . . .all friendships are based on the values two persons appreciate in common. . . .Deeper friendships arise when we can commune in the loves that we carry deep within us. . . .But the confirming element of friendship includes even more than loving the same things. There is also a delight in the uniqueness of the other, and this pleasure makes the loved friend more beautiful, bringing out his hidden loveliness. The true friend sees more in us than we see."[15]

Beginning with their exchange of prophetic greetings, in which Elizabeth recognizes Mary as "the mother of the Lord", and proceeding through to the conclusion of this three-month visit, we discover wholesome friendships blossoming in and around the Living God, their hidden unborn guest. These friendships are stamped as well by a certain Messianic urgency, a prophetic purpose fashioning a resolute solidarity amongst them.

The Birth of the Last Prophet: John the Baptist

The three-month visit seems to culminate on an extraordinarily positive note with the birth of Elizabeth's baby and subsequent days of joyful thanksgiving. (Luke's gospel does not indicate that Mary stayed for the birth of baby John, but it is assumed that Mary witnessed the event and then retold it to Luke; 1.57-80.) We can picture in our minds how Mary might have held the newborn John in her arms, kissing him on the forehead and softly whispering to him about her own little (unborn) baby, and the prophetic relationship they were destined to have in later years. "And her neighbors and kinsfolk heard that the Lord had shown great mercy to (Elizabeth), and they rejoiced with her. And on the eighth day they came to circumcise the child. . . ." (Lk 1:57-59).

More than nine silent months had passed before the birth and then another eight days afterwards. Zechariah was still unable to speak. Mary was preparing to leave for Nazareth, and now the final religious act would be celebrated to welcome the newborn baby and dedicate him among Abraham's descendants. An important chapter in salvation history was drawing to a close. What will the child's name be? Zechariah writes on the tablet; "His name is John." Fillion comments:

> For him, as for Elizabeth, the question was not open for discussion; the child's name had been chosen by a higher authority. Those present read this energetic reply, "and they all wondered." Not aware of what had occurred in the sanctuary, they did not understand why father and mother were in accord to derogate from the custom and choose a strange name for their son. The astonishment was at its height when (Zechariah) by a miracle suddenly recovered the use of his speech. "And immediately," says St. Luke, "his mouth was opened, and his tongue loosed." Having become dumb because of his lack of faith, he ceases to be so the moment he makes an act of obedience by giving his son the name prescribed by the angel. Consecrating to God the first fruits of his recovered faculty of speech, thus restored to him after a silence of nine or ten months, "he spoke, blessing God."[16]

Suddenly Scripture reveals to us the "real Zechariah" whom Luke had earlier described as "righteous before God". He is filled with the Holy Spirit; and now much older and much wiser than he was ten or more months before.

Zechariah's mouth, silenced for ten months or so, now breaks open, as though giving lyrical birth to a new creation of praise: "Blessed be the Lord God of Israel, for He has visited and redeemed His people, and has raised up a horn of salvation for us in the house of His servant David. . . ." The reader is encouraged to read this entire song (Lk 1:68-79).The canticle is dedicated to the coming of the Messiah: His meaning and impact upon Israel's destiny. "In only one sentence does (Zechariah) make mention of his son, John ('you, my child'). The rest of the hymn is taken up with thanksgiving to God for the great favor of redemption, which Mary's son is to accomplish. . . . .This scene is most vivid if we recall that the (Messiah) himself was present there, in his mother's womb. . . . . (Zechariah) shows, unlike many of the Jewish nation, that he understands the real purpose of Christ's coming: to save men from sin, not from the subjection to Rome."[17]

The canticle blesses God because "he has visited and redeemed his people". Note the word "visited" in the past tense. Unborn Jesus has been a visitor in Zechariah's house for three months. Yes, He has literally "visited" His people. But in fact the "visit" was not over; it was just beginning. The three-month visit of Unborn Jesus to the house of Zechariah the priest prefigures the three-decade visit of Jesus to the nation of Israel, with the birth of John pointing towards the new birth that lay ahead for the Chosen People.

While his hearers did not really understand what Zechariah was expressing, Elizabeth and Mary surely would.[18] He refers to the Messiah (hidden within Mary's womb, now about three inches in length/height) as "a horn of salvation" that has been raised up. How ironic that this symbol of God's strength and power should be used to describe such a tiny delicate infant, yet it is absolutely true. The "horn of salvation", we are told, is raised up in the house of David. This is obviously an explicit reference to "someone" other than the newborn baby John. As one bible scholar explains: "(Zechariah) and his wife were not descended from David. He alludes therefore, not to his own son, but to the Child of whom Mary was to be the Mother, in whom salvation was begun."[19]

The transformation in Zechariah's personal life is now complete. In his transformation from doubt to faith, sadness to joy, we witness the end of an age in Israelite salvation history. From B.C. (before

Christ) to A.D. (anno Domini; after Christ). As a priest he holds in trust the destiny of this priestly people, and in his transformation by God's faithful fulfillment of His promised Messiah, he represents along with Elizabeth the new creation in Christ: "From now on, therefore, we regard no one from a human point of view; even though we once regarded Christ from a human point of view, we regard him thus no longer. Therefore, if any one is in Christ, he is a new creation; the old has passed away, behold, the new has come" (II Cor 5:16-17). The "song" of Zechariah is testimony to this:

> A new heart I will give you, and a new spirit I will put within you; and I will take out of your flesh the heart of stone and give you a heart of flesh. Ezek 36:26

> Sing to the Lord a new song, his praise in the assembly of the faithful! Let Israel be glad in his Maker, let the sons of Zion rejoice in their King! Ps 149:1-2

With this final day of celebration Mary's extended visit now draws to a close. We can judge this first missionary and evangelical journey of the Unborn Lord and His Mother to be an overwhelming success. The visit concludes as it began, that is, with another inspired prophetic canticle of praise, like two bookends: Mary's "Magnificat" and Zechariah's "Benedictus". The former born of youthful enthusiasm, yet dwelling on the history of her people. The latter born of experience and age but focused on the future. Both are testimonies to God's merciful fulfillment of His promises to Abraham. Indeed, the "tender mercy of God" is the underlying message of these canticles. God's great mercy is a mystery, and as Mary, Elizabeth and Zachariah are learning, Unborn Jesus personifies and incarnates God's mercy. Unborn Jesus is mercy!

The Visitation Concludes

The Messianic joy that characterizes both the "Magnificat" and the "Benedictus" pervaded the three-month visit. But now Mary takes leave of the new parents and their newborn baby. Mary would have grown very close to Elizabeth and Zechariah during the course of these three months. And with the birth of John yet another strong bond was established between them all.

Previously we referred to Mary as the first Saint of the Incarnation. We have now met the second, third and fourth saints of the Incarnation – cousins of Unborn Jesus. The past three month visit is undoubtedly the most incredible "family visit" in the history of the world. (And the mutual love, friendship and respect characterizing the visit will seem all the more wondrous about six months from now when compared to the cool reception Unborn Jesus and His parents will receive in Bethlehem.)

As Mary says goodbye to Elizabeth, Zechariah and baby John with parting kisses, hugs and blessings, it is likely, as St. Bonaventure suggests, that Mary would have given a very special blessing to the prophet who was destined to "go before the Lord to prepare His ways..." (Lk 1:76).[20]

But we might surmise that the last blessing would have been given by the priest Zechariah to Mary, and more specifically, to her slightly swelling womb, wherein dwelled the Son of God, the singular hope for humankind. A heartfelt blessing, uttered from a stricken humility yet with staggering expectation.

CHAPTER FOUR ENDNOTES

1. Richard F. Clarke, S.J., "The Coming Of Christ", pamphlet D446 (London: Catholic Truth Society, 1964), 38.
2. St. Fulgence of Ruspe, "To Trasamund", *The Faith Of The Early Fathers*, Vol. 3, William A. Jurgens, ed. (Collegeville, MN: The Liturgical Press, 1970), 290.
3. Pope Pius XII, "*On Devotion To The Sacred Heart Of Jesus" (Haurietis Aquas)*, 1956, Heart Of The Savior, ed. Josef Stierli, trans. Paul Andrew, S.J., (New York: Herder And Herder, 1958), 233.
4. IBID., p. 231.
5. Mother St. Paul, *Ortus Christi* (London: Longmans, Green And Co. Ltd., 1921), 59.
6. St. Peter Julian Eymard, S.S.S., *The Real Presence* (New York: The Sentinel Press, 1938), 277.
7. IBID., p. 275-276.
8. "At 6 weeks of pregnancy, fetal heart pulsations can be seen on ultrasound beating at 125 beats per minute (bpm). By 7 weeks, the rate is 150 bpm, and at 8 weeks 175 bpm. By 16 weeks of pregnancy, the heart-rate has settled to between 120 and 160 bpm – about twice an adult's rate – which is the resting rate for the remainder of pregnancy." Stuart Campbell, M.D., Watch Me Grow (New York: St. Martin's Griffin, 2004), 37.
9. St. Ambrose, "Commentary On Luke", Christian Prayer: The Liturgy Of The Hours, (Boston: Daughters Of St. Paul, 1976), 1646.
10. Rev. L. C. Fillion, S.S., *The Life Of Christ*, trans. Rev. Newton Thompson, S.T.D. (St. Louis, MO: Herder Book Co., 1940), 253.
11. St. John Eudes, C.J.M., *The Life And The Kingdom Of Jesus In Christian Souls*, trans. by a Trappist Father in the Abbey of Our Lady of Gethsemani (New York: P.J. Kenedy & Sons, 1946), 196.
12. This paraphrase is not intended to be understood in a metaphysical sense.
13. David S. Yeago, "The Presence of Mary in the Mystery of the Church ", *Mary Mother of God*, ed. Carl E. Braaten and Robert W. Jenson, (Grand Rapids, Michigan: William B. Eerdmans Publishing Company, 2004), 72-73.
14. Could Zechariah hear while he was unable to speak? Some confusion arises because we read in Lk 2:62 that his neighbors and kinsfolk "made signs to (John's) father, inquiring what he would have him called". Why would they sign if Zechariah could hear? Two theories have been given. Perhaps they were speaking to Zechariah covertly, hiding their actions

from Elizabeth as they sought a second opinion. Or as Fillion suggests, when someone is signing to you (because he can't speak) you may be inclined to respond in kind (even though the individual can hear you); *The Life of Christ,* by Rev. L. C. Fillion, S.S., pg.275. Nowhere is it ever stated that Zechariah lost his ability to hear.

15. Ronda Chervin and Mary Neill, *Bringing The Mother With You* (New York: The Seabury Press, 1982), 22.
16. *The Life Of Christ,* by Rev. L. C. Fillion, S.S., p. 276.
17. Ronald Knox and Ronald Cox, *The Gospel Story* (New York: Sheed And Ward, 1958), 13.
18. We assume that the neighbors and kinsfolk gathered together for this celebration are ignorant of the fact that Mary is pregnant, just as we also assume that Joseph, family and friends back in Nazareth still don't know either.
19. Rev. C. C. Martindale, S.J., "St. John The Baptist", pamphlet (London: Catholic Truth Society, 1930), 13.
20. St. Bonaventure, O.F.M., *Meditations On The Life Of Christ,* trans. Sister M. Emmanuel, O.S.B. (St. Louis, MO: B. Herder Book Co., 1934), 25.

5

THE RETURN TO NAZARETH

As Mary takes leave of her dear friends, Elizabeth and Zechariah, and their newborn baby, her feet turn northward as her heart turns inward and heavenward. She recalls the wonderful birth of John, reliving the event, remembering excited faces and rejoicing, marveling at the beautiful little body of that baby. There is no treasure so precious and captivating as the small body of a newborn baby – old in months but new in the brilliance of daylight! Such "newborn joy" is contagious and – thanks be to God – not soon forgotten. (As Jesus said, the mother forgets her pain once the child is born [Jn 16:21]. So too, the family and friends of the mother and her newborn; they also are caught up in this new found newborn joy.)

Logically, Mary's thoughts lingered there to drink in and savor the message of encouragement and hope that this newborn baby – like every newborn baby – delivered to the expectant family. For this baby – like every baby – was a messenger from God, a messenger of peace. For truly it is one of life's great secrets: every newborn child is a witness to the Prince of Peace, and every birth day a little Christmas.

Eventually Mary's thoughts would have turned from the little baby John to her own tinier baby Jesus still growing within her. We can almost see her traversing a hillside descending on a beaten path towards the main thoroughfare, placing her hand upon her own womb where the Child dwelt calmly, peacefully. And now her own peace, increased by His Presence, shows upon her face in a knowing, thankful and hopeful smile.

Mary's Union and Identification with Jesus

She is the first Christian missionary. She carries the Christ across the land from this town to that. But He dwells within her – within and beneath her heart. The mystery of this particular heart-to-Heart, body-to-Body communion between mother and Child, Christian and Christ, is impossible to fathom. Many years later both Saints Peter and Paul described their own sense of oneness with Christ in words that may help us in our appreciation of Mary's experience. Reflecting on his own personal identification with Christ's death on the cross, St. Paul would say; "I have been crucified with Christ; it is no longer I who live, but Christ who lives in me..." (Gal 2:20).

But what of Mary's intimate identification with our Lord's Incarnation, the singular experience of Mary's maternity? Her sentiments may have resembled those of St. Paul; paraphrasing now: "I have been conceived with Christ; it is no longer I who live, but Christ who lives in me..." And as each day passed, did she not sense that she was becoming, as St. Peter would later say, a partaker "of the divine nature" (II Pet 1:4)? No other human soul has experienced the wonder and grace of this mystical passage from youthful human simplicity into the eternal mystery of mothering God! Words fail us here: " Christ is all, and in all" (Col 3:11).

Mary's Credo

Mary carries not only Christ within her, but also the original kernel of Christian doctrine and spirituality. She already holds fast to a Creed of Christian belief which is developing even as her Child develops within her. Her profound vision and grasp of her own Hebrew religion have laid the foundation for her faith. Her sources of this doctrine thus far are the angel Gabriel (sent by God to both Mary and Zechariah), Elizabeth, the unborn John, as well as Zechariah (all inspired by the Holy Spirit), and most directly, the Incarnate Word of God speaking within her.

The most recent installment of this Credo came through the prophesy of Zechariah which she must have recalled and repeated to herself now, letting the words play upon memory and heart together as a blessed melody but with a difference; this was a message from almighty God for her and for others. She realized even now she should remember these words of the Holy Spirit spoken through Zechariah and pray God to understand them (as she had previously committed to memory also the words of Elizabeth and her own "Magnificat"). She may well have smiled too recalling the last words spoken "...to guide our feet into the way of peace." She walked on peacefully, her Divine Guide within her, leading.

It was also clear to her now that baby John would later play a key role in the Messiah's life.

> And you, child, will be called the prophet
> of the Most High;
> For you will go before the Lord to prepare
> his ways... *Luke 1:76*

She had been struck once again to hear her unborn Child referred to as "the Lord". John would help her Son in some way. He was a prophet! What a great vocation God had planned for baby John. No wonder he had leapt when "the Lord" within her womb had first arrived. No words could describe the bond she felt with this family she had just left. The attachment she felt to baby John was particularly compelling and for the next thirty years – until his beheading – she probably remembered him daily in her prayer.

Twice in the second chapter of Luke's gospel we read that Mary "kept all these things... in her heart", referring to some unique events in the life of the newborn and child Jesus (Lk 2:19, 51). (Actually, this expression may well have been Mary's own words to describe the phenomenon.) Trustworthy and attentive as she was, Mary held on to all of her various experiences and teachings carefully, for safekeeping, treasuring them within her heart. The actions, the words, the meaning of all these things were there pondered and cherished. As Pope John Paul II once stated:

> You, O Virgin, found yourself placed at the
> very heart of these mighty works of God....
>
> You are the living memory of them.
> You are the Church's memory....
>
> Mother of the Incarnate Word!
> You are the human heart's immaculate sensitivity
> to all that is of God....[1]

And she, more faithful than the most diligent of scribes, carried this authentic creed of belief in Jesus, and would eventually share it with her husband Joseph. As Eve had shared the fruit and secret teachings confided to her by the serpent, so now Mary, the New Eve, goes to her betrothed with the fruit of her womb and of her heart – Jesus. Mary's humility, faith and obedience undo Eve's pride, lack of trust in God and disobedience. She is the true and living Ark of the New Covenant.[2]

Her Son's Prophetic Destiny

During the extended visit Zechariah would have frequently drawn her attention to various scripture verses concerning the Messiah. For Zechariah had been God's own scripture scholar, hand picked from all the priests of Israel to lead Mary through the scriptures so as to help her understand more deeply the awesome role of the Messiah and her responsibilities towards Him.

It seems not unlikely that, during the course of this prolonged journey by foot or donkey, Mary's thoughts would wander to Messianic scripture passages – searchingly, expectantly. Perhaps the strangest scripture passage of all, that is from Mary's perspective, would be from the book of Proverbs: "Who has ascended to heaven and come down? Who has gathered the wind in his fists? Who has wrapped up the waters in a garment? Who has established all the ends of the earth? What is his name, *and what is his son's name*? Surely you know!" (Prov 30:4, emphasis added). If ever there was a verse, a biblical riddle if you will, waiting for one person to answer it, this was it! Yes, she did know! An angel told her so.

Of course, Mary was familiar with most of the passages before Gabriel had even visited her, and on her own she was quite capable of wise reflection on these various prophecies. But nonetheless, she would have benefited greatly from this private tutoring by Zechariah.

Granted, we can not know the exact nature of Mary's thoughts and reflections in these circumstances, but we know she loved the scriptures and knew them well. They were alive for her! She was living out age-old prophecies. That is, she was physically, maternally linked to the One in her womb fulfilling all prophecy! To guide our reflections let's consider some of the Messianic texts from the Prophet Isaiah which were widely known throughout Israel.

Mary's thoughts would have flowed freely, uninhibited, for she knew that God was definitively intervening now in Israel – that the Messianic age was dawning – and there was a newness, a freshness, a cleansing about it all that was liberating. As Isaiah wrote:

> Then the eyes of the blind shall be opened,
> and the ears of the deaf unstopped;
> then shall the lame man leap like a hart,
> and the tongue of the dumb sing for joy.
>
> [As Zechariah had sung for joy at the birth of John the Baptist!]
>
> For waters shall break forth in the wilderness,
> and streams in the desert;
> the burning sand shall become a pool,
> and the thirsty ground springs of water;
> the haunt of jackals shall become a swamp,
> the grass shall become reeds and rushes.
>
> And a highway shall be there,
> and it shall be called the Holy Way... *Isaiah 35:5-8*

Indeed, here she was carrying the Holy One (Lk 1:35), and was not this very road she now traveled thereby made holy? The "Holy Way". Hadn't Zechariah spoken of baby John's prophetic role – alluding to the famous verse from Isaiah – "to go before the Lord to prepare his ways"? "A voice cries: 'In the wilderness prepare the way of the Lord, make straight in the desert a highway for our God'" (Is 40:3).

Decades later, after Pentecost but prior to the conversion of St. Paul, the early followers of Jesus were known as "belonging to the Way" (Acts 9:2). Here again we see Mary prefiguring the Church in a sense, even before the prophet John, she carries Jesus Who is the Way (Jn 14:6), across Israel, through wilderness, desert lands, countryside and villages. She blazes the first missionary trail and treads "a highway for our God": the Holy Way. By saying "Yes" to God, and by her faith and devotion she, too, is preparing – literally – the way of the Lord.

The Way of the Child Messiah

But there is another aspect of this "Way" which Isaiah also alludes to. Bible scholars today explain that chapters 7-12 of Isaiah form a distinct section – the Book of Immanuel – in which we find repeated references to the Messiah.[3] But within this "Book of Immanuel", there are a number of references to the Messiah as a baby and small child. This unique prophetic perspective on the Child Messiah would have fascinated Mary, and should be of great interest to our modern world. Let's consider some of these verses:

> Therefore the Lord himself will give you this sign: the virgin shall be with child, and bear a son, and shall name him Immanuel. *Isaiah 7:14* (NAB) [4]

> For to us a child is born, to us a son is given; and the government will be upon his shoulder, and his name will be called "Wonderful Counselor, Mighty God, Everlasting Father, Prince of Peace".... *Isaiah 9:6*

> The wolf shall dwell with the lamb, and the leopard shall lie down with the kid, and the calf and the lion and the fatling together, and a little child shall lead them. *Isaiah 11:6*

Isaiah, under the influence of the Spirit of God, focuses on a "child" (a son) who is the Messiah and more, he is Immanuel (God with us), Mighty God and Prince of Peace. And in some real way, this "little child shall lead" us. Not by mere coincidence has the Church come to love these prophetic passages with a tender passion. The Church sees the incarnational mystery revealed here in beauty, hope and peace.

Now if Isaiah was attracted by this "child", Mary was completely mesmerized. A shiver probably ran up her spine whenever she recalled the words: "...the virgin shall be with child, and bear a son, and name him Immanuel". For Mary was the virgin chosen by God to fulfill this prophecy and her unborn baby was the promised One.[5] But all Christians should share in that same prophetic shiver of anticipation at hearing "to us a child is born" and "to us a son is given". To us Unborn Jesus was sent as a sign of hope – and for every vulnerable unborn child: He is their only Hope.

Curiously, in this same passage from Isaiah we are once again given His "name": "Wonderful Counselor, Mighty God, Everlasting Father, Prince of Peace"! Actually these four words speak to the identity of this most special Child. Mary, the pregnant mother, would have meditated on these words often, perhaps recalling as she did, the singular Divine titles given to her Son by the Angel Gabriel, Elizabeth, Zechariah, and yes, even by the great prophet Isaiah! These witnesses unfold the Divine Identity of the tiny Person she carries within her womb. She was overcome by this reality – peacefully overwhelmed by the Prince of Peace.

No doubt her personal experiences in recent months gave her a new perspective on the various Old Testament prophecies. For example, the following image, also from chapter 11 of Isaiah: "There shall come forth a shoot from the stump of Jesse, and a branch shall grow out of his roots... In that day the root of Jesse shall stand as an ensign to the peoples; him shall the nations seek..." vs.1,10. Here is an image which parallels the prior references to the "child", showing first a shoot springing forth from the stump of Jesse, the father of King David, and then a branch from the root of Jesse. The shoot seems to become the branch: the shoot is like the early human development of the child who when full grown is represented by the branch. Admittedly, this symbolism would not be evident to most Israelites, yet it must have struck a chord with Mary: her body was nurturing this unseen living "shoot", the (unborn) "child", destined to save her people.

Among the prophetic images and signs representative of the future Messiah the image of this "child" is especially significant. Over two millennia of Christianity, the "child" has captured the hearts of the Christian faithful. Similarly, the attributes of this "child" in particular, and of all children in a way, have been a centerpiece of the Gospel message: "And calling to him a child, he put him in the midst of them, and said, 'Truly, I say to you, unless you turn and become like children, you will never enter the kingdom of heaven. Whoever humbles himself like this child, he is the greatest in the kingdom of heaven'" (Mt 18:2-4).

Jesus stood a little child in front of adults to illustrate the meaning of the kingdom of heaven. The childlike attributes He had in mind would certainly seem to include simplicity in belief, a matter-of-fact dependency upon God, a trusting faith in God and an innocent heart in one's relationships.

The Example of Unborn Jesus

On one occasion, when Jesus was preaching the Gospel message as an adult, he encountered a lack of faith. He looked up to heaven and called out: "I thank thee, Father, Lord of heaven and earth, that thou hast hidden these things from the wise and understanding and revealed them to babes; yea, Father, for such was thy gracious will" (Mt 11:25-26). This time, he did not employ children but babies to illustrate His point. Jesus Himself points towards infancy. Saint Josemaria Escriva once quipped in reference to "spiritual childhood": "Be little, very little. Don't be more than two years old, three at the most."[6] This half serious, half playful advice is thought provoking. There almost seems to be a progression here that suggests we not only become like children, but especially like "little" children, if not outright babies! And if trusting dependence upon God our Father is baby-like, then why not become as trusting as unborn babies?

Unborn Jesus was content to dwell serenely within the womb of His mother for nine months, trusting in God the Father and relying on both for His needs. In this He serves as an example for us. (Just as thirty years later He slept quietly in a boat during a turbulent and terrifying storm, so these two images show us how Jesus trusted God the Father during the everyday events of life, as unborn baby and adult.) This trusting attitude was tied to His complete confidence in the will of God the Father.

Unborn Jesus had been entrusted to His mother as every other unborn child is. Truly, in every unborn child within the womb we witness the epitome of entrusting one life to another. And every unborn child should enjoy complete security and peace within the womb of his or her mother, just as Jesus did. As Pope John Paul II observed, "The God of the Covenant has entrusted the life of every individual to his or her fellow human beings, brothers and sisters, according to the law of reciprocity in giving and receiving, of self-giving and the acceptance of others. In the fullness of time, by taking flesh and giving his life for us, the Son of God showed what heights and depths this law of reciprocity can reach."[7]

In his book, *The Son of Man,* Francois Mauriac begins with a chapter on childhood and, in a way, pledges his allegiance to childhood: "One part of our being, a most hidden part, is the child who has not experienced evil; by this fact a part of our being is like unto God. For God is not only a Father; He is also an Eternal Child...I put myself on the side of childhood...I am, above all, on the side of the Infant God who promised happiness to the meek."[8] When He came into the world as a tiny unborn baby, Jesus placed Himself squarely "on the side of childhood". He demonstrated His solidarity with all unborn children, and later with children at every stage of life. Would that all were pledged to be "on the side of childhood" – with the Infant God – throughout all of its many stages, from conception and early life in the mother's womb to late adolescence when the child prepares to go out on his own. If the world were truly on the side of childhood, we would live in a much more innocent and receptive world.

In Her Unborn Son Mary Had Hope

It is interesting to note that both Mary (in her "Magnificat") and Zechariah (in his "Benedictus") recall God's promise to Abraham and, in that light, see in their present situation the mercy and faithfulness of God. Quite possibly, as she now made her way back to her hometown of Nazareth, her thoughts turned for a time to her ancestor Abraham.

Had not the Lord made wonderful promises to Abraham? When Abraham was 99 years old, for example, the Lord appeared to him and said: "Behold, my covenant is with you, and you shall be the father of a multitude of nations" (Gen 17:4). And indeed, it had come to pass. But, Mary may have thought, these nations are not all serving the Lord, they are not all faithful to the God of Abraham, Isaac and Jacob. They are in need yet of restoration and healing... .the Messiah is their true hope now. And then, in the midst of thoughts such as these would not her heart have turned again towards the babe in her womb? Jesus, the Messiah. Unborn Baby Jesus, Hope of the Nations!

Destined to Suffer

By his writing tablet or through the kindly words of Elizabeth, Zechariah must have dutifully and tactfully, discussed some of the "suffering servant" prophecies with Mary as well. (Isaiah, in this series of four prophecies, foretells many of the sufferings of the Messiah; for example see Isaiah 53.2-11) Yet, it is likely that he didn't devote too much time or emphasis to these verses. They would have troubled her deeply and Zechariah would sense as much. And besides, it was not for him to speculate as to clouded meanings, perhaps inflicting unnecessary pain on the mother of the Messiah.

Such verses were probably the only sad point of her visit. Frankly, she wouldn't have liked thinking about them. But how could she avoid them entirely? Like a threat to the Child she was carrying, they may well have reared up and caused her sadness even now as she quietly traveled the byways of Israel. The greatest joy ever known to any human – her own present joy – was tempered by this one disturbing thought.

It might seem strange to say it, but in this respect, Mary was now beginning to suffer under the weight of God's redemptive plan and to be prepared by God for the trials ahead of her. Even now, three decades before the teaching ministry of Jesus, Mary is carrying her cross, within her heart, within her womb: the Christ! His Creed! Her Cross! (Many months later another old man inspired by the Holy Spirit, would authoritatively reveal to her the sorrow accompanying God's mission on earth, especially her own sorrow [Lk 2:34-35]....Further, she would flee Israel barely to escape a bloodbath arranged for her Son.)

But in contemplating thus, Mary's thoughts may have traversed the history of humankind, back to that first human couple and their tragic fall. Alas! She would recall God had already predicted conflict and suffering for her Son when He said to the serpent: "I will put enmity between you and the woman, and between your seed and her seed; he shall bruise your head, and you shall bruise his heel" (Gen 3:15). She was the woman (Jn 2:4 and 19:26). The tiny unborn Child within her was "her seed", the long awaited descendant of Eve who would do battle with the devil and triumph. Yet where such a momentous conflict would be played out, there would no doubt be suffering even to the Victor, as symbolized by the bruised heel.

Mary Anticipates Joseph's Dilemma

Reflections like these on the possible sufferings of her Son in the distant future would no doubt give way eventually to the "not so distant future" concerns which awaited her in Nazareth. Again, there was likely another nagging preoccupation, the practical matter of her betrothal and how her beloved Joseph would react to this unprecedented situation. She had an affectionate love for Joseph. Their relationship had a shy awkwardness about it because they were in love, they were betrothed to each other, but they were chaste and reserved in their expression of their feelings for each other. Nor had they had the opportunities for lengthy, private conversations. They knew each other, yet they didn't. They loved each other, yet they knew there was great room for an expansion of this love between them. They trusted each other implicitly but not based so much upon experience but rather, based upon a profound sense of the holiness and integrity of the other. Mary may have talked with Elizabeth – and maybe even Zechariah – about this "problem" of what to say or do. Even now she knew they would be praying for Joseph, as they all three had been during their visit together.

On the one hand, in justice she seemed to owe it to Joseph to forthrightly explain to him precisely what happened and then let him do what he would. On the other hand, this was God's plan not her's, and God had advised her and Elizabeth accordingly, why wouldn't God similarly reveal the matter directly to Joseph too? Most spiritual writers have assumed that Mary was resolved to pray for Joseph while remaining silent, waiting on the Lord.

There was no guarantee in Mary's mind concerning how Joseph would respond and so she proceeded now, as she would always, living by faith. As she approached Nazareth, what uncertainties and anxieties Mary may have struggled with regarding her own reputation and physical security, we do not know. But Jewish law provided harsh consequences for women suspected of adultery.[9] Mary understood quite well, that on a practical level, the key to her blessed predicament was in Joseph's hands. How would he respond? Nonetheless, one suspects that Mary had great confidence in Joseph as having been handpicked by God to be the earthly foster father to Jesus.

Perhaps as Mary drew near to her hometown, and now the hometown of her Son as well, she recalled the uncomplimentary saying of the southerners; "Can anything good come out of Nazareth?" (Jn 1:46) Again, she might have smiled or perhaps even laughed out loud as she considered a possible response; "Everything! Everything that the Lord ever promised to His people will come out of our beloved Nazareth!"

CHAPTER FIVE ENDNOTES

1. Pope John Paul II, Angelus Message, December 8, 1992.
2. While every mother is physically like a vessel or vehicle to hold, nurture and transport her unborn child, Mary's physical identity is more unique still given her extraordinary "passenger". She is the Ark of the New Covenant!
3. Charles F. Pfeiffer et al., ed., *The Wycliffe Bible Commentary* (Chicago: Moody Press, 1962) 607-621. See also Rev. Reginald C. Fuller D.D., Ph.D., L.S.S et al., ed., *A New Catholic Commentary On Holy Scripture* (Nashville and New York: Thomas Nelson, Inc. Publishers, 1979) 568-579.
4. *The New American Bible*, 1995-1996 edition, Fireside Bible Publishers, Wichita, Kansas, 67201.
5. Half of this prophecy is fulfilled now during the pregnancy and the other half will be fulfilled once the baby is born.
6. St. Josemaria Escriva, *The Way* (Princeton, NJ: Scepter Publishers, 1982) #868, 299.
7. Pope John Paul II, Encyclical Letter "The Gospel of Life" (*Evangelium Vitae*), 1995.
8. Francois Mauriac, *The Son of Man*, trans. Bernard Murchland (Cleveland,OH: The World Publishing Company, 1960), 17-19.
9. For a discussion of how Jewish laws and traditions dealt with marriage-related (betrothal-related) sins, such as adultery, see Henri Daniel – Rops, *Daily Life in the Time of Jesus* (New York: Hawthorn Books, Inc., 1962), 153-159.

6

Joseph Accepts Jesus as His Own Son

The New Testament begins with the genealogy of Jesus Christ through Joseph. Inasmuch as Jesus was in a thousand ways the fulfillment of all Hebrew Scriptures, it was most appropriate that Matthew set the stage for his gospel in this manner, linking the Savior with His own people and their profound history. This genealogy is also a good introduction to Joseph.

The genealogy begins with Abraham, "father" of the Hebrew nation and our "father in faith", and ends with Joseph the "father of the Savior". As Pope John Paul II explains:

> More important, however, is the genealogy of faith. . . .In this genealogy, this inheritance – an inheritance through faith – Joseph is inserted, the carpenter of Nazareth, the husband of Mary. Matthew's text shows us Joseph's faith at a crucial point in the history of salvation. As one time long before, Abraham had accepted in faith the message of God's saving promise, so too Joseph accepted the truth about that promise's fulfillment in Mary. He believed that she was "with child through the power of the Holy Spirit" (Mt 1:18). He believed as she herself, Mary, believed the angel's message at the moment of the Annunciation. . . . Thus Joseph believed and through this faith he not only entered into the great heritage of faith which has its origin in Abraham but, in the context of that heredity, fulfilled a call and mission which was totally exceptional, which was brought about around Mary and in her.[1]

After Abraham, came Isaac, then Jacob (and his son Judah). When Jacob was on his deathbed he gathered his twelve sons together around him and addressed them one at a time. To his son Judah he made the following prophecy: "The scepter shall not depart from Judah, nor the ruler's staff from between his feet, until he comes to whom it belongs;

and to him shall be the obedience of the peoples" (Gen 49:10). Twelve generations later we find the shepherd boy David (of the house of Judah) elevated to the position of King of Israel. However, the prophecy was not yet fulfilled.

At one point, King David told the prophet Nathan that he wanted to build a "house" (temple) for the Lord. But that very night God explained to the prophet Nathan that he wasn't interested in having David build such a house.[2] On the contrary: "Moreover the Lord declares to you that the Lord will make you a house....And your house and your kingdom shall be made sure for ever before me; your throne shall be established for ever" (II Sam 7:11, 16).

As centuries unfolded from King David to humble Joseph, the Lord's promise was reiterated by the prophets. "Behold, the days are coming, says the Lord, when I will fulfill the promise I made to the house of Israel and the house of Judah. In those days and at that time I will cause a righteous Branch to spring forth for David; and he shall execute justice and righteousness in the land" (Jer 33:14-15). Twenty-seven generations passed between King David and Joseph the carpenter. While he enjoyed lineage from David, it would not have occurred to Joseph, prior to his extraordinary dream, to think of himself as having any involvement in the coming of the Messiah. He was merely an uneducated carpenter from a small Galilean village. He knew something about building earthly dwellings but nothing about kingdoms and such.

That Joseph was a descendant of King David is an uncontested fact (see Mt 1:20, Lk 1:27,24 and the two genealogies of Jesus; Mt 1:1-17 and Lk 3:23-38). However, numerous theories abound regarding apparent divergences between the two gospel genealogies of Matthew and Luke. It is highly probable that Mary also was of King David's lineage (particularly if credence is given to the theory that the Lukan genealogy is through Mary rather than Joseph). Perhaps the most compelling scripture verse in support of Mary's Davidic lineage is Romans 1:3, which speaks of "...his Son, who was descended from David according to the flesh." [3]

Joseph's Betrothal to Mary

This simple carpenter seems to have been a rather quiet and deliberative soul. Nowhere in the Bible is there any record of Joseph speaking one word. Nor is there any reported instance of a one-on-one conversation between him and another person (even when he and Mary find the twelve year old Jesus in the temple – it is Mary who speaks). And very few of his actions are mentioned either.

His betrothal was a venturing out into a broader social world, embracing new relatives through marriage. With this betrothal a wonderful expansive joy must have begun to blossom within Joseph's heart. A quiet man confides little to others, but once he has confided his heart to one other, he becomes more open to heart-felt emotion and is freer to talk... at least with that one special other; she who holds his heart.

When Mary hastily left Nazareth did she speak with Joseph about her plans? Or was she too overcome to speak with him? Did she leave him a message? Or did Joseph escort her all or part of the way? We don't know. But we do know that they were in love, and that in her own way during this most extraordinary of situations, Mary took into account those treasured feelings and concerns of her beloved Joseph.

On the other hand, during Mary's three month absence, Joseph may have found himself in an unusual state of affairs. Here he is betrothed and his beloved quickly leaves town for three months. While not ranking as a village scandal, people may have wondered if there was some problem between Mary and Joseph. During this separation did she send word to Joseph of her welfare or visit? We don't know. Did Joseph go to visit Mary during the three-month period? Again, we don't know (but we might assume not, since Joseph had a living to earn, especially now with a marriage in the imminent future.)

Confined as they were by the limited communications of their era, yet they were both communicating with God through fervent prayer for one another. He for her well-being and she for his, but more – she prayed particularly for Joseph to discover God's Will in these unusual circumstances.[4] And no doubt, as the days for her return to Nazareth drew closer, her prayer – born of love for Joseph – grew more intense. And once she arrived in Nazareth who can imagine the heartfelt fervor of her prayer?

If the townsfolk hadn't wondered before Mary's return, some may have begun to wonder after. This is not to suggest that any confrontation occurred, but in a small community, absences, silences, and any unusual happenings tend to generate speculation and musings.

When Mary finally did return she would have been about thirteen weeks pregnant. She probably was not "showing", but she may have appeared to have put on a little weight. This early stage of pregnancy can be awkward if a woman starts to "look" slightly pregnant but hasn't yet revealed her secret. What happened next we don't know. Did other women in town notice her weight gain and jump to conclusions? Or did woman's biology linked with religious rituals betray Mary to other women in the village? [5]

Joseph's Agony

The Gospel of St. Matthew explains it succinctly: "... before they came together she was found to be with child of the Holy Spirit; and her husband Joseph, being a just man and unwilling to put her to shame, resolved to send her away quietly" (Mt 1:18-19).

This unspecified period of time – assumed to be sometime during the second trimester of her pregnancy – must have unfolded painfully for Mary and Joseph. Week by week the "obvious" grew more obvious. St. Bonaventure comments: "But she humbly kept silence and hid the gift of God. She preferred to be thought guilty, rather than to make known God's secret, and to say anything which would exalt her. She besought the Lord, that He Himself would deign to supply a remedy..."[6] And a twentieth century biblical scholar further elaborates: "But her secret was God's and she thought she ought not to reveal it without His authorization. Her faith and confidence told her, in the depth of her soul, that the Divine Spirit, who had miraculously informed the mother of John the Baptist about the mystery of the Incarnation, would likewise make it known to Joseph in due time."[7]

Assuming that Mary did not tell Joseph, nor even hint about what had occurred, we can not possibly know how it was that "...she was found to be with child..." Did Joseph come right out – albeit tactfully – and ask? What conversation transpired – if any – between the two about this matter remains unknown. Mother Angelica (of cable EWTN fame) sums it up this way: "He loved her too much and understood her too well to question her integrity, but he knew that the Child she carried was not his."[8]

What was Joseph thinking? Several Bible scholars have speculated:

> .... the plain facts spoke against her. If she had been the victim of some outrage, why had she not informed him?[9]

> The trouble is that it is as absurd to think that Joseph believed Mary guilty as to think that he did not.[10]

In Joseph we find a man who, in a matter of months, has gone from the heights of being betrothed to such a wonderful person as Mary, to the depths of resolving to send her away for such a reason. This was the extreme low point of his life! He had stepped out in faith and sought Mary's hand in marriage. In doing so he was taking one of life's risks, not knowing what might come of it. But in his wildest dreams he never would have imagined an outcome such as this.

No doubt during his life Joseph had looked to his namesake, the great Patriarch Joseph who had been sold into slavery by his brothers, as an example to follow (Gen 37-50). It may have occurred to him during these agonizing circumstances that the Patriarch had weathered similar tormenting events. He might have recalled how Potiphar's wife had falsely accused the Patriarch Joseph of attempting to lie with her, when in fact the exact opposite had been true and Joseph the Patriarch had fled from her.

Now Joseph the carpenter was facing a situation that seemed even more odd. Unlike the Patriarch, Joseph the carpenter was – in his own mind anyway – not in the position of being accused but rather in the role of a judge. Yet he was about to take leave, not of a temptress, but of his own most trustworthy betrothed. He faced not a dark prison with walls as had his namesake, but rather a dark cloud of tormenting confusion.

And in his own eyes, perhaps for a time, Joseph may have seen himself as a failure, maybe worse. He must have wept and mourned for the death of his marriage, his vocation, his holy dreams.

> I cry aloud to God, aloud to God, that He may hear me.
> In the day of my trouble I seek the Lord;
> In the night my hand is stretched out without wearying;

> My soul refuses to be comforted.
> I think of God, and I moan;
> I meditate, and my spirit faints.
>
> *Psalm 77:1-3*

But as we shall see shortly, Joseph was not only a man of deliberation but also a man of action. He reflected, prayed, and then he came to his decision. Many have speculated as to the reasoning of Joseph in his decision making. It seems sufficient to say that he did what he thought to be best in God's eyes and for Mary's well-being. In other words, not only was he a "just man", but he acted out of love in this difficult moment. Further, he conducted himself with dignity and treated Mary with respect, both in his thoughts as well as in his deeds.

The Annunciation of the Lord to Joseph

But just as God had intervened in the Patriarch's life through the use of dreams, so now God would directly intervene in the carpenter's life by the most wondrous dream ever:

> But as he considered this, behold, an angel of the Lord appeared to him in a dream, saying, "Joseph, Son of David, do not fear to take Mary your wife, for that which is conceived in her is of the Holy Spirit; she will bear a son, and you shall call his name Jesus, for he will save his people from their sins." .....When Joseph woke from sleep, he did as the angel of the Lord commanded him; he took his wife, but knew her not until she had borne a son; and he called his name Jesus.
>
> Matthew 1:20-21, 24-25

The unidentified angel addresses Joseph by the title "Son of David". (Many years later Jesus would be addressed by this same title.) In so doing, the angel seems to set the stage. The expression "Son of David" is a formal acknowledgement by the angel of the high dignity – might we say "office"? – being given to this lowly carpenter by Almighty God. Indeed, we have here the angelic equivalent, in the form of a title of honor, of that angelic greeting given to Mary months earlier; "Hail, full of grace, the Lord is with you!"

In Joseph's midnight angelic revelation John Paul II sees Joseph's "personal Annunciation" and the moment of his "Divine election....His place in the history of salvation is defined". The Pope, continuing his observations, points out that the response of Joseph was exemplary: "'When Joseph woke from sleep – we read in Matthew – he did as the angel of the Lord commanded him' (Mt 1:24). In these few words there is everything. The whole description of Joseph's life and the full characteristic of his holiness: 'He did'. Joseph, the one we know from the Gospel, is a man of action."[11]

Here then is Joseph's "fiat"! Mary's "fiat" was her total acceptance – in faith – of the divine will. Joseph's "fiat" was his immediate doing – in faith – of the divine will. Both of them demonstrate a vital faith stamped to its very core with the dual insignia: humility and obedience.[12] This radically sets them apart from the first parents, Adam and Eve, who thwarted the holy will of the Almighty, hiding from God in their cowardly confusion amidst the trees of the garden. Not only did God know He could count on Mary and Joseph, but He also knew where to find them.

Essentially the same message previously delivered to Mary was then delivered to Joseph. However, the annunciation to Mary by the great Archangel Gabriel was much more dramatic and detailed, involving a dialogue between the participants and concluding with a formal acceptance of the message delivered, whereas the annunciation to Joseph was merely one sentence spoken by an unidentified angel while Joseph was asleep. It would have been clear to Joseph that his was a supporting role to Mary. Accordingly, Joseph may have felt slightly "humbled" by this realization, or more than likely, he was such a simple and good natured soul that his realization was more one of thanksgiving for the privilege and honor extended to him than of weighing primary and secondary positions in the unfolding messianic plan.

Joseph fully cooperated with God's plan by his prompt obedience. On the surface this may not seem like such a great accomplishment. But in fact, this was the first of multiple angelic visitations (see also Mt 2:3-14, Mt 2:19-21 and Mt 2:22) and in every instance he was told what he should do, and he then did it. He had a one hundred percent performance record! Compare this with many of the great biblical figures or with one's own performance, and one realizes that such fidelity is rare. In Joseph's "no nonsense" example of committed obedience we find a fine model for all Christians. He is a man any son could be proud of, even the Son of Man.

The Fatherhood of Joseph

In a human and providential sense, God the Father wanted Joseph to "take His place" or "stand in" for Him during the gestation, birth and formative years in the hidden life of Jesus, before He grew into full manhood. This is an inscrutable mystery of divine logic which subtly reveals a divine plan providing for the well-being of Mary and Jesus, not just physically and materially, but at numerous social, familial, emotional, intellectual and spiritual levels as well.

From a legal and social point of view, Joseph would be recognized as the father of the baby Jesus. According to the Israelite understanding of marriage in those days, a child conceived during the time of betrothal was a "legitimate" child, and the reputations of both mother and child were thus protected. "Joseph's adoption of Jesus is effected in the two acts with which the account (Mt 1:24-25) closes, and which are in fact its most essential elements. 'He took his wife.... And he called his name Jesus.'"[13] This constitutes a turning point in the life of Unborn Jesus. His earthly father reaches out to Him, figuratively embracing Him with wholehearted acceptance.

The relationship between Joseph and Unborn Jesus becomes very real. Fr. Faber states that Joseph was "part of the scheme of redemption" and "assists God in keeping the mystery of the Incarnation a secret".[14] Joseph begins a secret "adoption" process while Jesus is yet an unborn child ("he took his wife" and her unborn child) and then the process is later completed with Joseph's naming of the child after birth and registering the child in Bethlehem during the census. Jesus needed to be accepted into a family, adopted into a family, and there existed a vacuum until that day when Joseph stepped forward in obedient faith to lovingly accept his son: "Joseph is the one whom God chose to be the 'overseer of the Lord's birth', the one who has the responsibility to look after the Son of God's 'ordained' entry into the world, in accordance with divine dispositions and human laws."[15]

When Joseph awoke from his dream and "took his wife" he now had an entirely new perspective on his life. He has just received two persons, two priceless gifts, and an assignment from Almighty God. Not gifts as possessions of course, but lives entrusted into his care. What a vote of confidence in one's abilities. The focus of his life is now his spouse, his child and the Messianic/Incarnation Mission – a joyful threefold blessing within his heart, a treble load upon his frail human shoulders.

In our study of Joseph thus far we have mentioned the awkward and even bewildering circumstances surrounding the conception, gestation and birth of Jesus. Are we not reminded of some of life's challenges confronting us today? Men can find in Joseph a noble and dignified model for responding to the mystery of each new human life as it makes its "ordained entry" into our modern world. By turning to God in prayer, for guidance and support, and by trusting in the Lord's promises and shouldering one's responsibilities, every man facing difficult circumstances should likewise find hope in the life of his unborn and newborn child. And also, others – grandparents, family members and friends – can all learn the profound truth about Joseph accepting this new human life. All those who are looking in from the outside, can find the blessing of solidarity with a new mother and her unborn or newborn baby.

It seems that it pleased Almighty God to show Jesus the love and protection of a human father and provide a male role model for Jesus (Jesus as infant, toddler, child, adolescent and young man). Joseph was a man Jesus could "look up to", a mentor He could study and learn from, a loving father He could confide in and trust. And judging by the life of Jesus as seen in the gospels, Joseph must have made an excellent contribution to the upbringing of his son Jesus.

It can be said that every boy needs a father. While cultures differ and customs change, a boy's need for an accepting father's thoughtful guidance does not. In those days, the father had a major role in the life of his son:

> It was the father who looked after his sons, and started to teach them his trade as early as possible....Education was also in the father's province....and as moral law merged into religious law, a father's first duty was to teach his children the commandments....In the same way, since the practice of religion and the history of the race both formed part of the Law, fathers told their children of all the wonders that Yahweh had done for His people; they explained the meaning of the great feast to them, and showed them how each of the customs that they observed had a holy significance.[16]

Similarly, there should be a husband/father at the center of each family. When Mary returned to Nazareth she was returning to Joseph, indeed, Joseph was probably the dominant reason for her return to Nazareth. With Joseph, there would be a certain earthly stability to their newly forming family. Throughout the pregnancy he was at work daily, keeping his small business running. There is no doubt that Mary came to depend and rely on Joseph, not only for the family's "daily bread" but also in a sense for direction. For example, Joseph received a total of four angelic dream encounters providing him with heavenly instructions for the well being of his family. Would these have occurred if he wasn't prayerfully receptive and sincere? In his dual role of husband and adoptive father Joseph supported the Incarnation Mission superbly. From the moment he was aware of God's wondrous plan, he strove to understand his responsibilities in relation to it and to honor these as best he could, always placing his wife and adopted child first. The Incarnation Mission of Unborn Jesus became Joseph's mission too.

And so the Father in Heaven wanted to be properly represented by a father on earth who would pass on to the infant Savior the Hebrew faith and heritage with integrity. Further, Joseph the tradesman, the laborer, would teach Jesus a work ethic which would be variously reflected throughout those later years of our Lord's public ministry when He labored tirelessly to build up the faith of Israel. It was part of the overall plan that the adult Jesus would be recognized first as a carpenter (Mk 6:3) and also as "Jesus of Nazareth, the son of Joseph" (Jn 1:45). And Jesus would later pass on this same work ethic – learned both from His Father in heaven and from His father on earth – to His disciples as He molded them into fishers of men and shepherds of souls.

The Mystical and Adoptive Fatherhood of Joseph

The fatherhood of Joseph is a great mystery. That is to say, that the fatherhood of Joseph – from the second trimester of this redemptive pregnancy onward – is a singular treasure of faith for the believer; and especially for adoptive parents and men of our own time. Too many have considered Joseph a mere family tree footnote; yet as we have observed thus far, he is so much more than that. Too many have given Joseph nothing more than an honorable mention at Christmas time. But we have now met the fifth faithful Saint of the Incarnation (chronologically speaking, not in order of importance). This is God's adoptive father. The question can legitimately be posed: "Has any man ever loved Jesus Christ with such a consuming and adoring love as did His own earthly father?" Here is one spiritual writer's observation regarding the significance of Joseph:

> He stood to Jesus visibly in the place of the Eternal Father.... The Human Soul of Jesus must have regarded him not only with the tenderest love, but also with deep reverence and an inexplicable submission. Meek and gentle, blameless and loving, as St. Joseph was, it is not possible to think of him without extreme awe, because of that shadow of identity with the Eternal Father which belongs to him and hides him from our sight even while it presents him to our faith. We cannot describe his holiness, because we have no term of comparison. It was not only higher in degree than that of the saints, it was also different in kind.[17]

Perhaps the point to be made here is that Joseph's singular role still has significance for individual Christians today. First of all, adoptive parents find a genuinely holy but down-to-earth model in Joseph. As Fr. Faber just pointed out, in relation to Jesus, Joseph stood "in the place of the Eternal Father". In a different order yet similar sense, the adoptive parent is chosen by God to stand in His place in relation to the adopted child. We can also compare him in a way, to Abraham or to the apostle Paul. Both of these men played unique roles in salvation history. Both held a "father-like" position in terms of their relationship to believers. The Jews of our Lord's time often referred to their "father Abraham" and Paul explained that in "faith" Abraham "is the father of us all" (Rom 4:16). But Paul also saw himself as a spiritual father to many others, such as the Christians in the city of Corinth (I Cor 4:14-17, also Phil.10). This is not about competing for loyalties however, as Paul rightly condemned in the same letter to the Corinthians (I Cor 1:10-13, 3:1-6). Rather, we are simply taking a cue from Jesus.

But what is unique about the fatherhood of Joseph? Many, many things. Let's consider its "adoptive quality". In chapter two we noted that with the conception of Jesus within the womb of Mary, the Mystical Body of Christ was also conceived. As Karl Adam put it, the Church "became objectively existent" at the moment of the Incarnation. We can also say that for the members of the Church, redemption was beginning and our adoption process as children of

God the Father – through Jesus Christ – was "objectively" underway, though far from completion. It was of course St Paul who explained that our redemption and adoption are linked mysteries of faith (Gal 4:4-7). But what the Eternal Father of Jesus was beginning mystically, the earthly father of Jesus was beginning physically. That is, while our redemptive adoption process was being initiated – through Jesus – even while Jesus was within the womb, so too the legal and familial adoption of Jesus by Joseph was also started. In a way, Joseph mirrors on the physical level a mystery that the Eternal Father has inaugurated on the spiritual level. A human adopts God and God adopts us.

Is it merely coincidence that Jesus was adopted before His birth by a human and now all humans are called to adoption through Jesus after His death? Can Joseph the father of Jesus, by extension, take on a unique comprehensive spiritual role or identity with respect to all of Jesus Christ's adopted brothers and sisters? Did Joseph perhaps represent all humanity when he adopted Unborn Jesus as his own Son? Or put another way, how are we, who are adopted through Jesus Christ, to relate to the one who first adopted Jesus Christ? [18] How remarkable and beautiful it is, that God chose to bring adoption into the center of the Incarnation mystery, and that the unborn baby Jesus was adopted by Joseph. The tender Heart of God is revealed here and all adopted children share in this unique experience with the child Jesus.

Finally, let's conclude our reflections on Joseph's relationship to Unborn Jesus by looking again to the Old Testament where we find all sorts of prophetic signs and types of things that are to come. Is Joseph the carpenter prefigured in the Old Testament in any way? Archbishop Alban Goodier answers:

> ....we do not wonder that anticipations are found of (Mary's) spouse, St. Joseph. Thus the faithful servant of Abraham, who brought Rebecca from Mesopotamia and protected her on her way; the faithful guardian Mardochai, who protected Esther, and directed her in her great task of saving her people; these and others would seem to foreshadow the Protector of Mary.
>
> But most of all is he seen in his namesake, Joseph, the son of Jacob and Rachel; and this anticipation would seem to be sanctioned by the Church in the free use made in her office of the story of one for the glory of the other. Joseph the dreamer: Joseph sent into obscurity in

> Egypt; Joseph unknown and unnoticed, though coming of a noble line; Joseph the spotless virgin, whose purity could not be sullied; Joseph entrusted with the care of a kingdom, so that "Go to Joseph" becomes the cry of hope for a whole people – one asks oneself of which Joseph these things are said, the old or the new, so perfectly does the type correspond with the antitype.[19]

"Go to Joseph" is what Pharaoh told the Egyptians when the famine struck and they cried to him for bread (Gen 41:55). Joseph the Patriarch was their provider for he was in charge of all the storehouses in the land. "Moreover, all the earth came to Egypt to Joseph to buy grain, because the famine was severe over all the earth" (Gen 41:57). In the Book of Psalms it is said of the Patriarch Joseph: "He made him lord of his house, and ruler of all his possessions..." (Ps 105:21). In a sense, God did for the carpenter Joseph what He did (through Pharaoh) for the Patriarch Joseph. God made St. Joseph the lord and provider to His Son, the Bread of Life (Jn 6:33-35) and St. Joseph brought Unborn Jesus to Bethlehem (this city name means "House of Bread") where Jesus was born, manifesting heaven's vast storehouses of grace.

Indeed, one wonders whether Jesus had His own father Joseph in mind, when He said to the people one day: "Or what man of you, if his son asks him for bread, will give him a stone?" (Mt 7:9) As a little boy, Jesus found He could rely on His father on earth in a way that reminded Him of His Father in heaven.

So we too, like Jesus, and like the hungry people of ancient days, can "go to Joseph" as to a kindly father and provider and ask him to pray for us. And he who heard the requests of his little boy in the bustling activity of his workshop, will no doubt hear the requests of God's children living today in this busy world of ours. And the fidelity of Joseph in all the matters entrusted to him reminds us – perhaps in a childlike way, as it reminded Jesus from time to time – how our Father in heaven is absolutely trustworthy in everything, always.

The Incarnation journey of Unborn Jesus gives us hope. By being trustworthy Joseph helped establish this initial context for Messianic and Redemptive Hope. So too, Christian fathers today must strive to be trustworthy, in both ordinary and extraordinary ways, and by their lives they can similarly bear witness to our Father in Heaven. And in family life we need to hear "go to father" and "go to dad" as words of hope and encouragement.

CHAPTER SIX ENDNOTES

1. Pope John Paul II, homily during visit to Archdiocese of Sorrento-Castellammare di Stabia, March 19, 1992.
2. Centuries later David's descendant, Joseph the carpenter, would literally build a small rustic wood house for the Lord to dwell in, though not exactly what the great King had in mind. And within that home he would have built – not a throne, but – a cradle and later a chair for the little baby Jesus.
3. The KJV translation is even more specific; "....which was made of the seed of David according to the flesh..."
4. One spiritual writer says that Mary prayed to Unborn Jesus for Joseph. Mary of Agreda, *Mystical City of God,* Vol.II, trans. Fiscar Marison (Albuquerque, NM: Corcoran Publishing Co., 1902), 315.
5. The Book of Leviticus, 15:19-30 instructs the people on the various ritual washings, cleansings and offerings linked to a woman's menstrual cycle. In the case of a pregnant woman the absence of all of these ritual acts would speak louder than words, particularly to other women.
6. St. Bonaventure, O.F.M., Meditations *On The Life Of Christ,* trans. Sister M. Emmanuel, O.S.B. (St. Louis, MO: B. Herder Book Co., 1934), 28.
7. Rev. L. C. Fillion, S.S., *The Life Of Christ,* trans. Rev. Newton Thompson, S.T.D. (St. Louis, MO: B. Herder Book Co., 1940), 282.
8. Mother M. Angelica, O.S.C., *The Promised Woman* (Birmingham, AL: Journey Into Scripture, Catholic Family Missionary Alliance, Our Lady of Angels Monastery, 1978), 18.
9. Fillion, *The Life Of Christ,* op. cit., pp. 282.
10. Jean Danielou, *The Infancy Narratives,* trans. Rosemary Sheed (New York: Herder And Herder, 1968), 40.
11. Pope John Paul II, General Audience, March 19, 1980.
12. In chapter one we identified the humility and obedience of Christ as being incarnational virtues – characteristics marking the Incarnation. Both Mary and Joseph were human models of these virtues in the way they both accepted and cooperated with the Divine will.
13. Danielou, *The Infancy Narratives,* op. cit., pp.45.
14. Rev. Frederick W. Faber, C.O., D.D., *The Blessed Sacrament* (Baltimore, MD: John Murphy Company, circa 1855), 188.
15. Pope John Paul II, Apostolic Exhortation Guardian of the Redeemer, trans. Vatican (Boston: St. Paul Books & Media, 1989), #8, 16.
16. Henri Daniel-Rops, *Daily Life In The Time Of Jesus,* trans. Patrick O'Brian (New York: Hawthorn Books, Inc., 1962), 127-128.

17. Rev. Frederick W. Faber, C.O., D.D., *Bethlehem* (Baltimore, MD: John Murphy & Co.), 131.
18. In the Dictionary of the Bible we are told that the original name "Joseph" (yosep) has two possible meanings: "let him add" or "let him gather". Curiously, through adoption, Joseph "added" Jesus to the Hebrew people and Jesus was formally "counted" during the census as one of us. And through the Son of Joseph we are all "gathered" into the Kingdom of God. John L. McKenzie, S.J., *Dictionary of the Bible* (New York, MacMillan Publishing Co., Inc., 1965), 455.
19. Archbishop Alban Goodier, S.J., *The Prince Of Peace* (Boston: Daughters of St. Paul), 34-35.

7

THE FIRST CHRISTIAN FAMILY

"....I bow my knees before the Father, from whom every family in heaven and on earth is named...."

Ephesians 3:14-15

If the Son of God had not come into our world we would not understand the Fatherhood of God, and if the Son of God had not been born into a family and lived so many years within His family we would not comprehend the full meaning of family life nor the compelling God-given mission facing every family.

Adam and Eve, Mary and Joseph, indeed every married couple will together create a family culture, establish and develop its family "name": identity, unique defining characteristics, emotional and intellectual traits, its own spirituality in relation to the Father in heaven. Discovering and building one's family identity is a work in progress best attempted with a healthy focus on God, faith and devotion.

The First Christian Parents

Their family "name" or identity is hidden and will have to be discovered by a married couple, just as the unborn child too is hidden, and needs discovery by the parents. For around the child the family grows to become what it was destined to be. In the case of Joseph and Mary, their family was centered around Jesus Whom they learned to discover and love, day by day, even before He was born.

Many diverse consequences come in the wake of the revolutionary Incarnation of God – a revolution of mercy. One of the major benefits was to the family as an institution, which was radically overhauled and strengthened from within, when this Divine Child entered into it. Redemption begins within the hidden recesses of Mary's womb. Redemption begins in the family.

Mary's pregnancy is one which brings renewal and reformation for from her womb the new family is born – the Christ-centered family. Recall that holiness and good will in the family of Adam and Eve were breached. The parents rebelled and their first-born son Cain – the world's first unborn baby – became a cold-blooded murderer. And so it went down through the ages. The family unit urgently needed rebuilding. In a remarkable way, God the Father reoriented and in effect, renamed the family, all families – past, present, future – when He sent His Son into this one.

> "At that time, says the Lord, I will be the God
> of all the families of Israel, and they shall
> be my people."...
>
> Again I will build you,
> and you shall be built, O virgin Israel!...
>
> 'The Lord has saved his people,
> the remnant of Israel.'...
>
> for I am a father to Israel....
>
> Jeremiah 31:1, 4, 7,9

The betrothed, and then married couple, Joseph and Mary can represent the "virgin Israel", and in their faithful obedience they represent "the remnant of Israel". Their family will become, as Jeremiah wrote, a prototype for "all the families of Israel," for within this family, the first, true Christ-centered family, there is one child alone, set apart, the Christ Child, and around Him alone humanity transitions from B.C. to A.D. Yale Professor and distinguished author Jaroslav Pelikan refers to: "....the teaching that the human birth as well as the divine birth was unique, so that He was the single and only-begotten Son of God but also the single and only-begotten Son of Mary – which meant that she was not only Virgin, but Ever-Virgin, as the Second Council of Constantinople decreed in 553."[1]

These first Christian parents are not parenting Christian children – rather they are parenting the Christ, the Son of the Living God. To say that their situation was unique is an absolute understatement. Their situation was foundational and definitive in terms of all the Christian families that would follow. As the original Christ-centered family, theirs was simple and straightforward in relational respects so that the character and mission of their family would be clear – like "a city set on a hill (which) cannot be hid" or a lamp placed on a lamp stand which "gives light to all in the house" (Mt 5:14-15).

Curiously, decades before St. Paul wrote his first letter to the Church of Corinth, Mary and Joseph had already reasoned – as the Messiah's parents and under the inspiration of the Holy Spirit – at least in essence, to some of the conclusions later enunciated so adamantly by Paul in that letter (see I Cor 7:1-40). (The reader is encouraged to read this section of the letter in the context of this reflection.) In this passage Paul is responding to practical inquiries he had received from this infant church. His detailed responses touch on almost a dozen different marital and single-life questions. He repeatedly makes the point about married persons having many worldly concerns which demand their attention as contrasted with those who "remain single as I do" (I Cor 7:8) and who are "anxious about the affairs of the Lord" (I Cor 7:32). Of course, there was nothing that Mary and Joseph wanted more than to "be anxious about the affairs of the Lord" in all the various stages of His childhood and adult life.

Paul also stresses that one should lead the life that God has "assigned" to him (I Cor 7:17), particularly the life that one had "at the time of his call" (I Cor 7:18). But the thrust of his message seems to be: "I wish that all were as I am. But each has his own special gift from God, one of one kind and one of another." (I Cor 7:7) No Christian ever had a more "special gift from God" than did Mary and Joseph. By abstaining from marital relations, and by being an otherwise childless couple, they could devote themselves exclusively to the One and only-begotten Son of God. Since the early centuries of Christianity the Church has taught that Mary conceived only one time, she had only one pregnancy and there was, of course, only one Incarnation. God knew how complicated we humans can make even the simplest of things, so He inspired the mother and adoptive father of Jesus to a single purpose and focus, to a most sublime single-hearted mission, similar to but very different from, the inspiration that St. Paul would later receive from the same Spirit. Most likely this inspiration was received and understood by them while Mary was still pregnant and they were still being prepared. In support of the redemptive plan, and by an act of free will, Mary did not have other children.[2]

Parenting the Unborn Christ Child

The Bible does not tell us exactly when Joseph took Mary and the Unborn Jesus into his home. But we know it occurred sometime after Mary returned from visiting with Elizabeth and Zechariah and before the family left for Bethlehem. We assume that it occurred shortly after Mary's return – sometime in the second trimester. Here we consider the approximate period of the second and third trimesters, that is, roughly the last six months of this pregnancy which changed human history.

Just as any "new" parents awaiting the birth of their first child are learning what it is like to be parents and planning ahead for the dramatic birth of their "firstborn", so too Joseph and Mary were learning and preparing. But for them there were many differences. They were taught by angels, by the Holy Spirit and by one another. For this was the Son of God, and as St. Thomas Aquinas wrote: "Mary and Joseph needed to be instructed concerning Christ's birth before He was born, because it devolved on them to show reverence to the child conceived in the womb, and to serve Him even before He was born."[3]

Shall we list among their parental responsibilities "the salvation of the world"? Not exactly. Yet somewhere between the age old duty of parenthood and their particular incomprehensible burden, they came to an understanding of their special call to be servants of the Lord. In a certain sense they even accepted this in a natural way, that is, with simplicity and true humility. So, like other parents their attention became focused – no, riveted – along with their spiritual life, on this unseen, unborn, unusual Child.

Like other pregnant women, Mary would have thought often about her own actions and their effect upon her unborn baby. When she ate and slept she was sustaining not only her own body but the little life within her as well. The larger she became, the more cognizant she was of her actions, and the more careful, lest she lose her balance and fall, thereby damaging the treasure within. Joseph too, as father and provider, could see in his own mundane actions – from repetitive work and household chores to the more personal and thoughtful actions to assist Mary – a supernatural service offered to One unseen.

All this by faith. They believed in the words of angels and they acted in accordance with this belief. Again St. Thomas explains: "But His first coming was unto the salvation of all, which is by faith that is of things not seen. And therefore it was fitting that His first coming should be hidden."[4]

Unborn Jesus: Resting, Recollected, Docile, Receptive

During much of the second and third trimesters, Unborn Jesus rested or slept – at times, perhaps up to "90 to 95 per cent of the day" – alternating perhaps between Eternal Peace and earthly distraction.[5] And for every unborn baby there is – or should be – a place of quiet refuge; hidden within the still womb of his or her mother. This concept is so engrained in the human psyche that in our culture it is recognized that there can be an undefined desire, midst the many troubles and pressures of life, to return to that original place of peace and safety; the womb.

Yet, in the metaphysical, spiritual and religious sense, God is our original and true refuge. The unborn baby within the protective, still and comforting confines of the mother's womb can represent this abiding in God our Refuge. More poignantly, the hidden Unborn Jesus is a model for us all of the docile and receptive soul: "Be still, and know that I am God…" (Ps 46:10) The womb is probably the quietest human habitat on earth; particularly when the pregnant mother is herself still. Rarely do we stop to think about the nature of stillness. Let us consider the serene existence of Unborn Jesus and our own stillness as well. (And for the present purpose we will orient these reflections to our stillness in rest, sleep and death.)

There are many different ways to "rest" and to understand this concept – the key to it is found in the Commandment: Remember the Sabbath day, to keep it holy (Ex 20:8).

Other passages from the Book of Exodus further elaborate upon the rationale of this command:

> It is a sign for ever between me and the people of Israel that in six days the Lord made heaven and earth, and on the seventh day he rested, and was refreshed. *Exodus 31:17*

> Six days shall work be done, but the seventh day is a Sabbath of solemn rest, holy to the Lord... *Exodus 31:15*

We see then, that this Sabbath day is "holy" and that in some mysterious way God was "refreshed" by resting on it. For us too it is holy and for our "solemn rest", which no doubt, will be refreshing to us also. As the book *Prayer in Practice* explains: "Behind this seventh day, therefore, there is the mystery of God's rest. God's rest, not man's rest, is the meaning of Sunday, and from the former the latter derives its justification. Man must open himself to this significance.....On working days man is bound by duty; on the seventh day he is free."[6]

Sunday is meant to be a day of refreshing liberation from the worldly matters of toil and work. A day of renewing oneself. To collect one's thoughts – that is, to pick up the pieces of one's life dropped during the past six days – to collect oneself, and to recollect oneself. And additionally, it is a time of preparation for the next six days.

Is it possible that by contemplating the "resting" of Unborn Jesus in the womb of His mother that we might learn yet more about God's resting? In some manner can we partake of or unite ourselves to, God's resting? Caryll Houselander addressed this question:

> In Advent Christ rested in Mary – still, silent, helpless, utterly dependent. The Creator trusted Himself to His creature....This was a foreshadowing of what the Incarnation would mean for us; for in us too, Christ rests as He rested in Mary. From the moment when the Christ life is conceived in us, our life is intended for one thing, the expression of His love, His love for God and for the world....We must allow the Christ-life to grow in us in rest. Our whole being must fold upon Christ's rest in us, as the earth folds upon the seed.[7]

So Christians can unite themselves to Jesus and His resting and thereby perhaps better appreciate God's rest. The unique St. John Eudes wrote many diverse prayers during his lifetime demonstrating his desire to offer every action of each day to God in a special and meaningful way. This is reflected in prayers such as this: "O Jesus, I offer Thee the rest I am about to take, in honor of the eternal rest Thou dost enjoy in the bosom of Thy Father, and in honor of the sleep and temporal rest Thou didst take in the bosom of Thy Mother, as well as during Thy whole life on earth."[8]

His reference to the "bosom of Thy Mother", is an endearing term for the womb of Mary as we see in the following instruction he gave elsewhere to retreatants: "Your retreat ought to be made with these chief ends in view: 1. To continue and honor the various retreats of Jesus, for example, His retreat from all eternity in the bosom of His Father; His retreat for nine months in the bosom of His Mother..."[9] During his times of rest, sleep and even retreat John Eudes was reminded of Unborn Jesus within Mary's womb. As he instructs us above, we can honor these acts of Jesus to the extent that we join ourselves to Him with these mysteries of His Presence in mind.

Sleep is similar, yet different. When one thinks about one's sleeping – enveloped within the covers of the bed, the room darkened, sounds silenced, action ceasing, senses quieted, thoughts slowly leaving the mind – one realizes that these hours of sleep are unlike any other hours of the day. In fact, perhaps when we sleep we come closest to re-enacting our earliest months of life within the womb. In this sense we recognize the restorative and healing aspects of night time sleep: "In this unnerving darkness is set the gift of sleep, a gift because we have to receive it without any exertion, without any taking, we have only to let it come. The night is God's daily reminder that we are creatures with many limitations who can stand even sanity only so long and must after sixteen or seventeen hours of it give up."[10]

Sleeping through the night – like Sunday rest – is really a time of transition from one day to the next. Similarly our Lord's nine months within the womb of Mary was a time of transition; from being eternally begotten to being temporally begotten. But in the transition there is also preparation, as Ronald Knox wrote:

> Almighty God has given us, for the ordering of our lives, an alternation of day and night. "Each day echoes its secret to the next, each night passes on to the next its revelation of knowledge." The day by its brightness typifies his glory, the night by its darkness recalls to us the profundity of his mysterious being...And so our life is marked out for us by alternations; each day is separated from the last by a thick black line of oblivion....And meanwhile, this alternation of day and night has served another purpose; it stands to us for a model and a sacrament of human life in general. As the darkness

> closes round us, we go through a dress rehearsal of death; soul and body say good-night to one another; and the soul wanders off into that unreal country where it can neither sin nor merit, can neither miss nor grasp opportunities. And then morning comes, and with morning, a re-birth. Each day, then, begins with a birth and ends in a death; each day is a life in miniature.[11]

As the body, mind and heart seek peace in rest and sleep, and ultimately find it through death, so the soul seeks God its refuge in stillness. And in a sense we find refuge from time when we sleep and die. And how similar the womb is for the unborn child in transition, between eternity and earthly destiny; a reassuring refuge. And in Unborn Jesus, there was a singular, fuller expression of all these mysteries of life.

The Adoration and Prayer of Unborn Jesus

> *". . . pray to your Father who is in secret; and your Father who sees in secret will reward you."*
>
> Matthew 6:6

The first secret place of prayer known to our Lord was the womb of Mary. As many spiritual writers have explained, Jesus in the womb of His mother enjoyed secret communion with His Father. Fr. Faber considers this topic and attempts to:

> .....construct a biography of the Eternal Word during those Nine Months in Mary's Bosom. His chief and sovereign occupation was in adoring God......in the first moment of the Incarnation, not only were the amazing decrees of everlasting wisdom fulfilled, and creation with incredible magnificence completed, but the creation thus completed turned round as it were to the Face of the Creator, and worshipped him with a worship equal to himself......He saw reasons we can never see for adoring God......This was his incessant occupation. All other occupations centered in this, resolved themselves into this, and identified themselves with this. It is the single occupation, of which the rest are manifold developments. Hence also, as we shall see hereafter, he occupied himself with rejoicing in his created nature, and not least of all because, by its seeing God clearly, it possessed such an idea of worship, which the Hypostatic Union gave him the capabilities of satisfying.[12]

In His adult years Jesus had many out-of-the-way places for prayer; in the wilderness (Mt 4:1), a lonely place outside of Capernaum (Lk 4:42, Mk1:35), a wilderness place in the region of the lake of Gennesaret (Lk 5:16), in the hills of Judea (Lk 6:12), the Garden of Gethsemane on the Mount of Olives as "was his custom" (Lk 22:39-41) and no doubt many others. And so it was not surprising that while instructing his followers on prayer He made a point of emphasizing the importance of privacy and solitude: "But when you pray, go into your room and shut the door and pray to your Father who is in secret..." (Mt 6:6). But where did this habit of solitary prayer begin? Perhaps His father Joseph – quiet Joseph, who is never quoted once in the Bible – provided this example. But before His childhood, within the chamber of His mother's womb He began, in an unfathomable fashion, to worship and pray.

> The Word took possession of her chaste womb, where He was to dwell for nine months – the first nine months of His sojourn on this earth. And in that temple He at once began His work, that of loving God with a human heart......All His perfect acts of love, of praise, of reverence, of service, His acts of patience and humility, of meekness and suffering, of sacrifice and mortification – and all the rest, passed up to God through Mary. From that sacred temple a fragrant incense was continually rising to heaven – "a sweet-smelling savor", sweeter than either earth or heaven had ever known before. For all those acts were perfect in God's sight, worthy of His acceptance; they were the acts of a perfect man. And they were also infinite because they were at the same time the acts of God Himself.[13]

In the previous quote by Mother St. Paul, she refers to the work of Unborn Jesus as "loving God with a human heart". This interesting choice of words reminds us that this is also our primary work. She goes on to flesh out the nature of the communion between the Unborn Son and the Heavenly Father. The Son's acts are heart-born and Heart-directed, and draped in prayer appropriate to the unique incarnational circumstances.

A Life of Prayerful Solitude

Prayer is a force which can change human lives and the destinies of nations. Prayer – childlike or mystical, pleading or praising, offered in fear or thanksgiving – if heartfelt and humble, is unrivalled in its influence and transforming capabilities. How then are we to understand the worship and prayer offered by Unborn Jesus? Father Faber explains: "Worship alone is power, intellectual power and moral power, the power of world-wide change and of all beneficent revolution. We not only learn this lesson from the life of confinement which the Incarnate Word led in Mary's Bosom, but it is that life which gives our life power to become universal like itself."[14]

In studying the worship and prayer of Unborn Jesus we can also glimpse from afar the life of the Trinity; a rich subject for contemplation. Father Faber wrote: "Now this life in the Bosom of the Father seems to devout souls made visible, intelligible, and familiar to them by our Lord's life in His Mother's Womb, and is the chief reason of that most interior devotion."[15]

Unborn Jesus subtly demonstrates several basic qualities of a fruitful prayer life. In stillness He is recollected and ready for God, His human activities are worship-filled and adoring towards His Father, He is receptive to the will of God whether marvelous or mundane and His Spirit is docile. He is the original model par excellence of a spirituality that is obediently childlike. While the womb environment was only temporary and very confined, yet we see here the foundation for His later prayer life during childhood and adulthood.

They Magnified the Lord Together

As mother – biologically, genetically, emotionally – Mary was becoming progressively more and more attuned and sensitized to the growing, thriving life within her. Yet something greater had been taking place within her soul which would have enormously affected her thoughts, affections and prayers. She had developed a kind of spiritual rhythm in her daily living which was not her own doing. The life within her had His own spiritual life, and while His physical body was very tiny, His spiritual presence far outshone her own and she felt completely dependent upon Him, and further, strengthened and guided by Him.

The presence of God Incarnate within her was actually redefining her spiritual life. She now relied less on her own mind and heart to lead or steer her. Now, with a veritable fountain of grace springing up within her, she was compelled to "think" less and simply "adore" more. She who had been accustomed previously to letting God take the lead, was now even more ready to let the Son of God within her, re-shape her life, not just physically but in every way.

We might say that during the nine months He spent in her womb, our Lord was subtly teaching Mary about the spiritual life and prayer. This being so, and inasmuch as Mary is for us a model of the interior life, we could claim that, in a sense, it is the Unborn Christ Child who exemplifies the very life of prayer.

> He, in her, carried on the blessed converse with His Father; there was never any separation between Mary and the Blessed Fruit of her womb, Jesus. She would come back to Him with all the more joy, and tell Him what she had been doing and saying...When we think of Jesus praying for nine months to His Father, when we think of Mary's nine months' colloquy with Jesus, we begin to think that there is something wrong about our methods of prayer, that they need re-modeling. Let us try to understand something of what His prayer was.[16]

The normal physical movements of the unborn child during the second and third trimesters are very aggressive at times. In fact, the unborn infant in this buoyant environment of amniotic fluid is frequently more active than after he or she is born. (Although once the unborn infant becomes too large for the confined space of the womb, in the last few months of pregnancy, his body is more restricted and hence less active.)

The unborn Jesus would have been no exception. Week by week He would be discovering new movements of which He was now capable. Whether reaching, grasping, jumping, swimming, thumb sucking or whatever, He would experiment just as other unborn infants would. These adventures of earliest infancy which were once yours and mine, were His as well.

Mary would have begun feeling the "quickening" sensations within her own body around the fourth month. As the months progressed, Joseph could have also witnessed the outward jabs of small fists punching and pushing, or feet kicking, elbows aimed sideways. There is every reason to imagine that Jesus was a normally boisterous infant in the womb, and that His antics delighted Mary and Joseph.

Even the senses of the unborn Christ Child were developing, and sudden loud noises in Joseph's workshop – such as hammering – may have been the first distinct sounds He heard coming from beyond Mary's body.[17] Likewise, He would have felt heat on those occasions when Mary might have been cooking or working close to a hot fire. His dreaming while asleep in the womb – as all unborn babies do – would have been inspired in some fashion by such simple experiences in utero. In adulthood, we know that He was a sound sleeper (as when He slept in the storm tossed boat, Mt 8:24). With a little imagination we can picture the unborn infant Jesus sleeping peacefully within the womb of His mother contentedly waiting for nature to catch up with Him.

Even the physical movements of her Son within her womb, which she could feel, and later even partly observe from without, were as signs of the more profound spiritual and intellectual movements of the soul of Jesus. For His part, Jesus too was experiencing the sense of touch as He would touch the inner wall of Mary's uterus via the thin veil of the amniotic sac. This divine touch within from within – one can almost envision a Sistine Chapel-like ceiling painting of God, not the Father but the little unborn Son, straining forward and reaching out His tiny finger towards the inner heart of Mary His mother – can almost give shape to God's way of touching each human heart from deep within. There was a continuous exchange between mother and Child, not only on the physical level but at every level. As the book *To Jesus Through Mary* states:

> . . . .as in the natural order, the thoughts, ideas, impressions, etc., of the mother are transmitted to her unborn child – and this in an unfallen state, might have been greater than at present – so Our Lord, coming into this world a little infant, and showing, too, how great was His desire to be as other infants, would take from His Mother what other children take from their mothers; that is to say, He would wish the same influence exercised upon Himself while unborn that is exercised upon other unborn children by their mothers.[18]

Nonetheless, in this particular mother-Child exchange it was the Child Jesus who was the dominant participant, and His mother was the frequent recipient to the extent that Mary's life was a reflection, a magnification of the hidden, unborn Divine Life within her.

There are many perspectives on the nature of the mother-unborn child relationship. One doctor, reflecting on the commandment "To honor your father and mother," says that this should really be a "reciprocal relationship of honor". In this light we can appreciate all the more the dignity of this special relationship between Mary and her unborn Child Jesus. "From the moment of conception, through gestation, to birth, and beyond, the mother must honor her child. . .even as the child, in an incipient way, honors his or her mother by a trusting dependence on her, by learning her voice, her heartbeat, her moods, and her goings about, all of which he or she will remember after birth."[19]

Finally, let us not forget that Joseph too, though a latecomer to this communion of hearts, would have been quickly caught up in the spiritual tempo of it all and would have followed Mary's example of adoring and magnifying the unborn Divine Presence. So we find in this Holy Family, a trinity of hearts united peaceably, and of One Will.

The First Christ-Centered Family

There is a biblical account of how Moses one day helped the people of Israel in battle by standing atop a high hill with his hands uplifted. But when he lowered his hands because of weariness the tide of the battle changed unfavorably, so he sat on a boulder and Aaron and Hur were on either side of him holding his hands up for him all day long 'til sunset. His people won the battle decisively (Ex 17:8-13). This image of one person being helped by two others on either side of him to change the course of history is a wonderful image. Truly it is an image of the support parents together offer their child.

Similarly, Joseph and Mary lived their lives around Jesus Who was the very center of their family. As parents they would give Him every support they could, for the battle of redemption was already underway. And so they stood at His side every day, even when He was yet unborn, to hold Him up in this initial stage of His mission. And indeed, thanks be to God, from the moment of His Incarnation the tide of this supernatural battle, this battle of battles, began to turn, and His parents faithfully carried out their specific duties in this regard.

What Jesus would later teach His followers we see lived out in this first Christian family: "For where two or three are gathered in my name, there am I in the midst of them" (Mt 18:20). These words of

Christ the Lord were literally and physically true with respect to His family life. Both Joseph and Mary were "gathered together" with Unborn Jesus. Every minute of every day, He was in their midst.

The image referred to earlier of Moses with hands outstretched is relevant in several ways with respect to Mary and Joseph. Not only did they support the Christ Child parentally on the natural level, but He supported them continually as well. Christ in their midst, with outstretched arms – outstretched horizontally as when crucified and/or lifted triumphantly as when raised from the dead – in a sense reverses the image and lifts up the arms of His parents in prayer, supporting them supernaturally and otherwise. And with regards to the day-to-day routine of marriage, even the monotony of it at times, we discover here the secret of the Christ-centered marriage: "Thou dost show me the path of life; in thy presence there is fullness of joy..." (Ps 16:11).

While every child brings an indefinable joy to marriage, Christ brought a continual, unceasing, supernatural joy to it beyond all expectation! So in the case of Mary and Joseph, their daily life in Nazareth even before the birth of Jesus, was punctuated by prayer and this profound joy – joy of the Lord! In this exact manner, their marriage is a model for every marriage. This first Christ-centered family is a model for every family and for the Church community as well.

The Unborn State Is Sanctified by Unborn Jesus

By coming into the world as a little unborn baby, and living that existence for nine months, Jesus sanctified the unborn state and the relationship between the unborn child and his parents, particularly the relationship with his mother. Day after day, month by month Jesus was nothing but an insignificant unborn baby. He chose this restricted unborn life to show the depths of God's love for us. Perhaps the world can not understand nor appreciate it, but we Christians must!

The modern world would have us judge unborn babies superficially by our limited abilities of observation; what we can observe them doing, learning, achieving and mastering. Not so with God. He sees us for who we are, rather than what we can or can not do. As the philosophical maxim states; "action follows being". When God appeared to Moses He revealed His identity by stating: "I AM WHO AM." So too, it is more important that we discover Who Unborn Jesus is rather than what things He might have done as an unborn baby.

And the same is true for all unborn babies. God designed "personhood" to be a secret core mystery of life to be discovered by oneself and others on nature's terms, not ours. God hides the "unborn person" in the womb, almost in a suspended state of love – that is, suspended between God's creative love for the new creature and the mother's nurturing love – until the beauty of the infant's physical development is sufficient to reflect the fullness of the infant soul. As one professor of pastoral theology has noted "awe is intrinsic to parenting".[20] Months of waiting contributes to the sense of awe that parents experience through pregnancy and birth. And awe is also an essential element in respecting human life as both gift and blessing.

Parents who, respecting nature and nature's God, patiently wait for the birth of their child, grow themselves in that very virtue – patience – that they will need most in the upbringing of the child. The "unborn person" is literally a "buried treasure" of personhood and personality but, like wine, needs to age. Such a respectful attitude was that held by Mary and Joseph during the months of the second and third trimesters. It should be the attitude of all expectant parents.

CHAPTER SEVEN ENDNOTES

1. Jaroslav Pelikan, "Most Generations Shall Call Me Blessed: An Essay in Aid of a Grammar of Liturgy", *Mary Mother of God*, ed. Carl E. Braaten and Robert W. Jenson, (Grand Rapids, Michigan: William B. Eerdmans Publishing Company, 2004), 8-9.
2. The traditional view of Mary as "Ever-Virgin", that Joseph and Mary did not have marital relations, is not only held by Catholics and Orthodox Christians, but by many others as well. For example, Martin Luther held this position and forcefully argued it in a treatise entitled CHRIST WAS BORN A JEW – "The Christian in Society" II, *Luther's Works*, Vol. 45, Helmut T. Lehmann et al., ed. (Philadelphia, PA: Concordia Publishing House and Muhlenberg Press, 1962), 212. "....Zwingli, and other Reformers insisted that Mary remained a virgin even after the birth of Jesus. This view was endorsed by Bullinger and inscribed in the Second Helvetic Confession (1566), one of the confessional documents in the *Presbyterian Book of Confessions*." Daniel L. Migliore, *"Woman of Faith", Blessed One*, ed. Beverly Roberts Gaventa and Cynthia L. Rigby, (Louisville, KY: Westminster John Knox Press, 2002), 119. Regarding gospel references to the brothers and sisters of Jesus (Mk 3:31, 6:3, John 2:12) Martin Luther argued that this terminology was commonly used to include cousins and other relatives. Indeed, there are clear examples in the book of Genesis of these terms being used as such, and even today in some cultures this practice continues.
3. St. Thomas Aquinas, O.P., *Summa Theologica*, III, Q. 36, art. 2, ad2.
4. IBID., III, Q. 36, art. 1, ad 3.
5. Stuart Campbell, M.D., *Watch Me Grow* (New York: St. Martin's Griffin, 2004), 87-88.
6. Romano Guardini, *Prayer In Practice*, trans. Prince Leopold of Loewenstein-Wertheim (London: Burns & Oates, 1957), 30-31.
7. Caryll Houselander, *The Passion of the Infant Christ* (London: Sheed and Ward, 1949), 22-23, 15.
8. St. John Eudes, C.J.M., *The Life and the Kingdom of Jesus in Christian Souls*, trans. by a Trappist Father in the Abbey of Our Lady of Gethsemani (New York: P.J. Kenedy & Sons, 1946), 122.
9. IBID., p. 281.
10. J. Neville Ward, *Five For Sorrow Ten For Joy* (Garden City, N.Y.: Doubleday & Company, Inc., 1973), 40.
11. Rev. Ronald Knox, *A Retreat for Lay People* (Harrison, N.Y.: Roman Catholic Books, 1954), 23-24.

12. Rev. Frederick W. Faber, C.O., D.D., *Bethlehem* (Baltimore, MD: John Murphy & Co.), 76, 70-71, 76.
13. Mother St. Paul, *Nativitas Christi* (London: Longmans, Green and Co. Ltd., 1937), 145-146..
14. Faber, *Bethlehem*, op. cit., pp. 73.
15. Rev. Frederick W. Faber, C.O., D.D., *The Blessed Sacrament* (Baltimore, MD: John Murphy Company, circa 1855), 168.
16. Mother St. Paul, *Ortus Christi* (London: Longmans, Green and Co. Ltd., 1921), 90-91.
17. Ironically, one of the very last vivid sounds the adult Jesus would hear just prior to His death, would be that familiar hammering sound, this time of nails being driven through His hands and feet.
18. Mother Mary Potter, *To Jesus Through Mary* (New York: Catholic Book Publishing Co., 1960), 118.
19. Dr. Joseph H. Hagan, "Reflections On Pope John Paul II's 'Letter To Families'", L'Osservatore Romano (Vatican City), August 31, 1994, p.7.
20. Bonnie J. Miller-McLemore, "Pondering All These Things", *Blessed One*, ed. Beverly Roberts Gaventa and Cynthia L. Rigby, (Louisville, KY: Westminster John Knox Press, 2002), 109.

8

Sent by God to Bethlehem

In those days a decree went out from Caesar Augustus that all the world should be enrolled. This was the first enrollment, when Quirinius was governor of Syria. And all went to be enrolled, each to his own city. And Joseph also went up from Galilee, from the city of Nazareth, to Judea, to the city of David, which is called Bethlehem, because he was of the house and lineage of David, to be enrolled with Mary his betrothed, who was with child.

Luke 2:1-5

In a worldly kingdom a ruler wants to know the names and numbers of the peoples he rules. How many mouths to feed, how many to serve or manipulate, how many to protect and how many potential soldiers to conscript. And, of course, how many taxpayers!

Now the Roman Empire prided itself in its worldly accomplishments. It was a vast civilization, sprawled out across the earth, yet maintaining law and order within its borders, law by military power and order by uniformity, government organization and communications. So a census would be a typical governmental exercise to further the interests of this worldly state.

As the people of Israel heard of the decree and generally were resigned to obey it, we see this chosen people being called – by a gentile – to go back to their ancestral roots, back in time so to speak; to trace their lineages back through their "fathers" to their cities of origin.

In a way time would stop, or at least history would pause for a short period, industry would be curtailed, the roads in between villages filled with Israelites returning to their family's city. Human history's deformed flow was for a short time arrested so that the Empire's inventory could be taken.

But of course there is a superior ruler to all earthly ones: the Lord of Heaven and earth. And the Lord would use this worldly bureaucratic exercise for much loftier ends. From the divine vantage point, it could serve as a reminder to the people who, as they made their way back (physically) to their fathers' cities, might travel otherwise in their hearts and minds back to the days of their fathers, and perhaps even back further to that one true place of origin – the Garden of Eden – and recall that their first allegiance must always be to the Father-Creator. Yet unlike Caesar, their Creator already knew how many they were. At least. . .it might give them pause.

More importantly, Caesar is unwittingly setting the world stage for the entrance into human affairs of the world's Redeemer. This Redeemer, as yet unborn and unknown, returns not to His Father's heavenly city, rather He has just come from there. He comes to confound the Roman Empire's census, to elevate it if you will, to skew the results by being counted among them. He is more than a mere statistical saboteur, for once they have counted God as one of themselves they will be caught in a most merciful divine plot, planned high above the clouds with the ultimate and final heavenly census in mind, in which all people will be counted and separated, like sheep and goats, by the Eternal Shepherd (Mt 25:31-46). Yet, He will be the least of all those counted in Bethlehem, a stranger to that town and region, newborn and tiny, utterly helpless, almost unnoticed, almost not counted.[1]

Of What Value, This Child?

Luke 2:1-5 refers to an "enrollment" being held throughout the Roman Empire, but of course there are a number of ways to translate the original Greek. Other possible meanings might be "registration" or "taxation". It is likely that this "census" actually served several purposes. Not only would the people be counted, but their land holdings would be registered and their buildings and major assets would be assessed for taxation purposes. An enrollment of this type would be very ambitious:

> A Roman commission, aided by Jewish-Herodian collaborators who knew the country and language, would move through the land and remain a few months in each locale....every plot of land, every house had to be assessed. Witnesses had to be interrogated, disputes settled, etc....Those people who had property rights there journeyed there to validate these rights for themselves and for their children, and to oversee their evaluation and to assure that their taxes would not be set too high. Only those people were involved who, like Joseph, had rights in their birthplace, be they in the form of possessions, rents from possessions, or inheritances....Joseph doubtless had many reasons for this decision. In the first place he knew that the expected child was a holy one and since he could give this child the rights of the Davidian house, it was not only in his own interest but also in the interest of the child that he represent these rights....This child would be Joseph's heir, and in consideration of this the father acted conscientiously and with the utmost solicitude.[2]

It is curious to contrast the purely materialistic ends of the Roman census with the spiritual realities that unfolded in conjunction with it. The mundane and material would be transformed into the glorious and supernatural. As an unborn infant en route, Mary's unborn child had no status within the Roman Empire, yet once born, He would have a legal identity.

So then, one Jesus of Nazareth was destined to be counted along with all of his countrymen. What belonged to Caesar would be given to Caesar; this head count. But of infinitely greater significance was the fact that what belonged to God would be given to God by virtue of the newborn Redeemer; countless hearts, previously discounted, in Israel and throughout the world.[3]

As at the end of His life, when Pontius Pilate would have the name of Jesus formally inscribed and posted at the top of the cross, so at His birth, Caesar would note for public record the singular name of baby Jesus (newborn son of Joseph of Nazareth, carpenter).

The Holy Family Living the Fulfillment of Prophecy

Now the question can be posed; "Prior to the proclamation of Caesar's decree, did Mary and Joseph have any reason to think that the Messiah would not be born right there in their home town of Nazareth?" It is likely that they did. The Gospel of Matthew quotes the great prophecy of Micah (5:1-4). Probably Mary and Joseph recalled this prophecy. Even if they did not recall it of their own accord, it is probable that Zechariah had mentioned it to Mary during her visit to his home. Yet, with every prophecy there is also ambiguity. So, while it might have seemed to them that Bethlehem was likely to be the birthplace of the Messiah, it was not necessarily completely clear that it would be.

Mary and Joseph understood too that the scripture emphasized the prophetic and historical relationship between King David and the coming Messiah. As St. Thomas Aquinas would point out a thousand years later, King David was born in Bethlehem but set up his throne and the temple in Jerusalem, similarly, Jesus too was born in Bethlehem and would consummate His Kingship and Priesthood in Jerusalem.[4]

We can picture Mary, now in the final trimester of her pregnancy, perhaps working at home or on an errand out in the town center, when she suddenly hears the news – a census decree by Caesar requiring Joseph and her to travel to Bethlehem. A wave of joy and relief breaks upon her soul as she sees God intervening not only in her life, not only in the history of her own people, but with one universal sweep of His Almighty Hand in the history and destiny of the entire world! She is in awe, realizing that yet another prophecy is to be fulfilled – not abstractly or disinterestedly, as some "head count" might be – but intimately in her own life, in her own person and body and family, in the city of David.

> But you, O Bethlehem Ephrathah,
> who are little to be among the clans of Judah,
> from you shall come forth for me
> one who is to be ruler in Israel,
> whose origin is from of old, from ancient days.
> Therefore he shall give them up until the time
> when she who is in travail has brought forth;
> then the rest of his brethren shall return
> to the people of Israel.
>
> Micah 5:2-3

The words of this prophecy could now be more fully appreciated by four Israelites; Mary, Joseph, Elizabeth and Zechariah. Particularly the more obscure words – "whose origin is from of old, from ancient days" now held a remarkable meaning. God's Son, eternal like God His "Father"; together their origin reaches back through time, beyond time's beginning, into some old ancient unknown "days" before days were defined or numbered, before the earth existed. Eternally uncreated! (As the Nicene Creed states: "...eternally begotten of the Father, God from God, Light from Light, true God from true God, begotten, not made, one in Being with the Father.")

Based on her astonishing experiences thus far and those words of the prophet Micah, Mary understood that her pregnancy (and unborn child) was different from all other pregnancies: a constant mystery of faith to her. This pregnancy of her's had been the subject of prophecy, explained in scripture; angels had come to earth to reveal its holy hidden meanings. Her baby, in some sense existed before King David was conceived, before Abraham was called. As her now unborn child would explain it thirty years hence: "Truly, truly, I say to you, before Abraham was, I am." (Jn 8:58)

She would probably also have considered at length Micah's words; "... when she who is in travail has brought forth..." Mary knew that this prophecy, these exact inspired words, referred specifically to her, and were linked to the "little" town of Bethlehem. Like pieces of a puzzle the information was being handed to her as she needed it, one piece at a time, and joined together so that with each revelation her fathoming of the Divine Plan was all the more profound. And her time was quickly approaching.

The Third Journey during the Redemptive Pregnancy

The census decree was for Joseph and Mary a Divine Decree, and so they prepared to leave Nazareth on their prophetic journey towards the long-awaited event. It would be about a ninety mile journey and given the advanced stage of her pregnancy they might only average about ten or fifteen miles per day. So the trip there would take about a week, but how long would they be away? For months perhaps, or maybe longer? Most likely Joseph brought some of his carpentry tools with him so that he could support himself and his family as needed.

Their neighbors and friends must have foreseen the possibility of the birth occurring en route or in Bethlehem. Practical presents of clothing for a newborn baby may have been brought to them as they prepared to leave their hometown. Mary would have carefully packed these along with swaddling cloths or other items which she had probably made. As the couple took leave of family and friends, their donkey loaded down with various compact staples, they could never have imagined – not in their wildest dreams – what experiences lay ahead of them. All was in God's hands, as God was in theirs.

As she had right at the outset of her holy pregnancy, once again now at the very conclusion of her pregnancy, Mary again sets out on a journey towards a small town on the outskirts of Jerusalem. This, the third "evangelical" journey of her pregnancy, was distinctly different from the prior two (the first to Elizabeth's home, the second back to Nazareth). Joseph was now a central character in this Messianic mission. And she was now only weeks, or maybe days away, from delivering her baby and fulfilling many age-old prophecies.

Carrying the Son of God within her, she was supremely confident, and with Joseph at her side she was consoled and comforted along the way. Obviously the interaction between Mary and Joseph on this journey is something we know little about.[5] To the casual observer the two weary travelers would have appeared inconspicuous and unimpressive. Yet they are parents to God's revolution of Love, the first pair of (adult) disciples to be sent out "two by two" (Lk 10:1) bearing (literally speaking) the Good News; the Word made Flesh. They foreshadow the endless stream of all missionaries whose footfalls would turn the entire globe into mission lands after hearing each his or her own call: "As the Father has sent me, even so I send you" (Jn 20:21).

The One Who Sends Is Also the One Who Leads

In an Advent meditation Mother St. Paul considers how Unborn Jesus shows Himself to be a Leader:

> He it is Who though as yet hidden is nevertheless leading all.....He it is Who is now leading the whole world and placing everybody in his own city. He it is Who is leading Joseph away from Nazareth. He it is Who is leading His own Mother over every step of that difficult and tiring journey, letting the joy in His own Heart overflow into hers; and He is my Leader too. With such a General, nothing will be overlooked in my life; everything will be arranged in wisdom and love.....Oh! come, little Leader, come and redeem us.[6]

The prophet Isaiah had said that in the Messianic age; "... a little child shall lead them..." (Isa 11:6). During the Christmas season we reflect on this and other joyous prophecies, but we don't often think of Jesus before His birth as being directly involved in the fulfillment of any of these prophecies. But He was. Even though hidden and unseen He was truly present and active! He was "the Way" before birth as well as after. Here, along the road to Bethlehem He leads the Way for us to follow.

It was prophesied that He, shepherd-like, would lead the sheep. Unborn Jesus was to Mary as an "inner voice"; the voice of the Good Shepherd, the very voice of God! He was leading not only Joseph and Mary, but many others even then before they reached Bethlehem His birthplace. For example, by supernatural means He used a natural phenomenon – a "star in the East" – to lead wise men from the East, to meet Him as by a specially arranged appointment after His birth. So, as three of the Chosen People (Joseph, Mary and Unborn Jesus) make their way southward toward Bethlehem, also on another road westward three heathens were heading toward this convergence of cultures, beliefs and the fulfillment of Heaven's plans and prophecies which would occur at Bethlehem. Bethlehem – crossroads of the world! As Father Faber wrote, the unborn Jesus is not only leading, He is also approaching.

> The nine months draw to a close, and our Lord's last act is to journey from Nazareth to Bethlehem. It is toward us, as well as toward Bethlehem, that He is journeying. He is about to leave His home a second time for the love of us. As He had left His uncreated home in the Bosom of the Father, so is He now going to leave His created home that He may come to us and be still more ours. He will show us in this last action that He is not obedient merely to His holy and chosen Mother, but that He has come to be the servant of our commands and to wait upon our forwardness....[7]

The Obedience of Unborn Jesus and His Parents

The obedience of Jesus to the will of His Father in Heaven is the common theme running throughout the entire course of His earthly life; from His conception to His Ascension into Heaven. Mother St. Paul underscores this point:

> Think of His obedience in the womb of His Mother. His very Incarnation was an act of obedience. He waited for Mary's Fiat. His waiting nine months was purely an act of obedience to the laws of nature..... All the time that He lived in Mary, He obeyed all whom she obeyed – St. Joseph, the Roman Emperor, the people at Bethlehem. He gave up His own Will to others. This was His method of being zealous. This is how He did the work that He had come to do. Can I adopt this method? It is not easy..... If my zeal for God is to be worth anything, let me follow the methods of God Incarnate in the womb of His Mother and be absolutely obedient to God, to His Holy Church and to those whom I ought to obey.[8]

To understand obedience as Jesus understood it requires a joint effort of intellect and will so that thinking on it we would then live it; as St. James once stated: "But be doers of the word, and not hearers only..." (Jas 1:22). Obedience of this magnitude originates from the depths of an altogether unfathomable humility.

In fact, Jesus is the source for this teaching about the spirit of humility and obedience. One example is the following: "... whoever would be great among you must be your servant, and whoever would be first among you must be your slave; even as the Son of man came not to be served but to serve, and to give his life as a ransom for many" (Mt 20:26-28). Elaborating upon these sentiments St. Bede (673-735 A.D.) relates this notion to our Lord's submission to the census: "He deigned to take flesh at such a time that, shortly after His birth, He would be enrolled in Caesar's census, and thus submit Himself to bondage for the sake of our liberty."[9] This concept of servitude and slavery as a key spiritual teaching is something rarely discussed today. This is probably due, in part, to the brutal political realities of forced slavery, particularly when tied to prejudice and racism, as it has been witnessed in the not-too-distant past.

St. Paul makes a number of references to himself as a slave of Christ the Lord. These are referenced here because it is very possible that Mary and Joseph, before Paul's time, also had this sense of being slaves or servants to God's will generally speaking and, more particularly to the Messiah Who was their son. In both Rom 1:1 and Gal 1:10 Paul sees himself as "a servant of Christ" (RSV). In the Knox translation; "a slave of Christ". But in I Cor 9:19, both RSV and Knox translations (and other translations) use the term "slave" when Paul says:

"For though I am free from all men, I have made myself a slave to all, that I might win the more."[10]

Now returning to the topic of this journey undertaken by Mary during her last month (or weeks) of pregnancy, we can picture the weariness she must have endured. The journey must be undertaken, but she makes it carrying a (human) burden – her unborn Son. She is yoked with Him, inseparable. They are yoked by organs; they each have a distinct organ specifically for this mother-child bond; the uterus (mother) and the placenta (child). Of course, Mary is not a grumbler, a moaner, a whiner, or a complainer like many of us. Unselfish love makes this burden more than bearable, rather it is desirable. She lived what her Son later taught His followers: "Take My yoke upon you, and learn from Me; for I am gentle and lowly in heart, and you will find rest for your souls. For My yoke is easy, and My burden is light" (Mt 11:29-30).

She has been carrying her burden many miles over the past nine months. But as she approaches Bethlehem, she prepares herself for the delivery of her burden. Actually, only in part, for she carries this holy burden both in her womb and in her heart. So while the physical burden will be delivered, the spiritual one, previously conceived in a sense, will be both carried and delivered all her life. She who carries our unborn Savior now along the dusty road southward will be called "blessed" for all generations.

The Longsuffering of Unborn Jesus

Many prophecies abound in Old Testament scriptures concerning the Messiah and the Messianic age that was to come. One of the less palatable prophecies is that of the suffering servant. Isaiah spoke in vivid terms of this one who would come to serve God on behalf of the people of Israel and suffer dearly for it (and in Handel's "Messiah" His lot is portrayed memorably with wrenching, soul-tormenting tones). Let us pause and consider for a moment the suffering unborn servant, on the road to Bethlehem: "...like a lamb that is led to the slaughter, and like a sheep that before its shearers is dumb, so he opened not his mouth..." (Isa 53:7). Are we being overly dramatic here? Billy Graham once put it this way: "He had taken on a human body in order that He might die. From the cradle to the cross, His purpose was to die."[11]

So here on the road to Bethlehem He is being transported – in one sense unwillingly, by government dictate – to meet with His destiny as a Victim to be offered for the sins of the world (albeit thirty years hence). This mystery of the Savior's suffering servant (slave) identity, even before birth, caused John Donne to say to Mary, in his Holy Sonnet, Annunciation, that Unborn Jesus: "...yeelds himselfe to lye in prison, in thy womb..."[12] And here follows yet another reflection upon this progression from unborn suffering servant (slave) to unborn criminal, as though serving a sentence of nine months in an inhospitable jail cell:

> Consider the painful life that Jesus Christ led in the womb of his Mother, and the long-confined and dark imprisonment that he suffered there for nine months. Other infants are indeed in the same state; but they do not feel the miseries of it, because they do not know them. But Jesus knew them well, because from the first moment of his life he had the perfect use of reason....The womb of Mary was therefore, to our Redeemer a voluntary prison, because it was a prison of love. But it was also not an unjust prison: he was indeed innocent himself, but he had offered himself to pay our debts and to satisfy for our crimes. It was therefore only reasonable for the divine justice to keep him thus imprisoned, and so begin to exact from him the due satisfaction. Behold the state to which the Son of God reduces himself for the love of men, he deprives himself of his liberty and puts himself in chains, to deliver us from the chains of hell.[13]

I confess to the reader, that when I first read the above quote by the prolific author St. Alphonsus de Liguori (1696-1787), I thought it to be rather negative, if not morbid. But as I reflected upon the pathetic state of our world with the practice of legalized abortion-on-demand commonplace across the globe, I realized that God alone had foreseen such a day when all unborn babies would be regarded with suspicion and their lives in jeopardy.[14] The two authors just quoted, who perceived Unborn Jesus as a kind of prisoner in His cell (womb), lived during historical periods when abortion was illegal and rightly considered immoral. Seeing Jesus in this light was somewhat prophetic in the sense that, unbeknownst to them, at a future time – that is, now in our own sad time – the unborn would be treated like criminals, or rather, worse than criminals! (Criminals are generally granted fair trials and continue to have basic human rights even while in custody. Not so with unborn babies.) The unborn child has almost no rights at all in most countries at the time of this writing.

Our Savior shared in the sufferings of today's unborn little ones! Anticipating their persecution, He had them close to His tiny Unborn Heart and "set (His) face like a flint" towards Bethlehem! Who could have ever, in their wildest imaginings, conceived of such a thing as an unborn baby criminal? Only God could foresee that such an irrational period in human affairs would one day arise. And so the Unborn Savior began carrying the cross of all unborn "convicted criminals" long before His birth in Bethlehem; before Herod's troops were unleashed in a ruthless baby hunt!

> *There is no end of it, the voiceless wailing,*
> *No end to the withering of withered flowers,*
> *To the movement of pain that is painless and motionless,*
> *To the drift of the sea and the drifting wreckage,*
> *The bone's prayer to Death its God. Only the hardly, barely prayable*
> *Prayer of the one Annunciation.*[15]

The Unborn Christ and the First Christian

The journey to Bethlehem is almost done, we climb steeply now to a rise in the road from which we look back and see a series of divinely orchestrated events and forward to holy promises which will soon be fulfilled. We come to this point in the story of Unborn Jesus, when His birth is mere days or weeks away. We step back for a moment and wonder, "How will the world learn of all these early events in our Lord's life, those that have already occurred and those that are yet to unfold in Bethlehem, Jerusalem, Egypt, Nazareth and thereafter?" The Church will hear of them from the first witness to Jesus Christ – His mother. The foundation of the Christian faith will be built upon the Incarnation of the Son of God. But by whose testimony do we believe "that Jesus Christ was conceived by the Power of the Holy Spirit"? There is no record of Jesus telling anyone this explicitly. His mother told the early Church about the story of His Incarnation and they believed. Thus, we too believe!

Mary would not have spoken of these things until the Holy Spirit led her to do so. And when she did speak, it would be about Her Son:

His Life, His Mission, His story. (Just like an Icon in the tradition of the Orthodox Church, we can picture Mary with Jesus in her arms, and she is pointing to Him.)

To better understand the collaboration between Unborn Jesus and His mother, we need to focus briefly, not on the "person" Mary, but on the predestined prophetic role she was called to. For example, consider that within the short span of 27 verses at the outset of Matthew's Gospel, five different Messianic prophecies relating to Mary and her baby are quoted and said to have been fulfilled: Mt 1:22-23, 2:5-6, 14-15, 16-18 and 23. By whom are they fulfilled? Primarily by Unborn Jesus and His mother, newborn Jesus and His mother (and adoptive father Joseph). Here are the prophets whose prophecies are fulfilled: Isaiah (7:14), Micah (5:2), Hosea (11:1), Jeremiah (31:15) and Isaiah (11:1). All goes according to God's plan from "before the foundation of the world" (Eph 1:4).

By being pregnant Mary is fulfilling Isaiah's prophecy. The mere fact that they are now on the road to Bethlehem is part of the fulfilling of Micah's prophecy. And so it goes. By virtue of her maternity, Mary was drawn into a spiritual orbit round the Incarnate Word of God within her. He, like the sun and she like the dependant planet earth, are in a relationship that goes beyond simplistic analysis. Together they fulfill ancient Messianic prophecies; He in the primary role as Savior, she in the secondary dependant role as Virgin Mother. His is the leading role – a role no mere mortal could play – hers is the first supporting role which, by divinely predestined design, turns out to be an indispensable one.

Mary became the living link between the Old Covenant and the New Covenant, between B.C. and A.D. She was the foothold in our human time-line where God alights, Incarnate, to change human destiny. As she lives this Incarnation transition she is herself transfigured by it. She becomes, by heavenly design, the "one-of-a-kind" collaborator with Jesus – His first disciple, the first member of the Mystical Body of Christ – the Church.

Mary was chosen and instructed by God to shoulder these awesome responsibilities. With God's help she committed to memory all of these events and revelations – treasuring the words – reflected upon them and prayed about them.[16] But these are not merely stories and conversations that she is dealing with, rather, this is the original subject matter of a primitive Creed of Faith; faith in Jesus Christ and His New Covenant. The Church would build the central doctrine of Christianity – the Incarnation of the Son of God – upon the testimony of Mary. A rock solid trustworthy testimony, like that foundation Jesus later spoke of, upon which to build one's house or life (Mt 5:24-27). With penetrating insight Lutheran professor David S. Yeago says of Mary, that she:

> ....is not simply a biophysical vessel, an unwitting conduit...her pregnancy is located within a context of covenant and communion, of God's election and promise and the faith that these evoke...Mary is not simply a private person but a public one; she is called by the angel's proclamation to an office, a public role within the communion of God's people and the history of God's salvation...her bodily "bearing" of Christ is inseparable from her faith."[17]

Mary, the mother of Jesus lived each step of these foundational Gospel events with Jesus. So that we might believe it, she lived it, remembered it, pondered it, treasured it, and finally at the proper time shared it. No other Christian has carried within themselves, for a lifetime, such sacred experiences and Divine Revelations surrounding the mystery of the Incarnation of God, while these actual mysteries – as historical, yet profoundly personal events – were still occurring. As John the Baptist was the precursor of the Messiah, so Mary became the precursor of the Church. And as John prepared the way of the Lord, Mary prepared the way of the Christian believer, by living each Christ event with her Son, trusting God all the while.

Mary has, in a sense, two pregnancies. On the one hand she is literally pregnant with Unborn Jesus while on the other hand, she figuratively carries within her heart – in its embryonic and developing stages – the Gospel of Jesus Christ. She has taken this elemental Christian Creed to heart, along with her Savior, and lives her every day according to this one faith only. Unborn Jesus is her child and her doctrine! Not only is she championing the Incarnation mission of Jesus Christ, Mary herself has become the first champion of the Christian faith!

So the Incarnation is not only Christ's story (God's story), but it is also Mary's story (that is, humanity's story). No wonder then that it is so dear to each one of us! For weak and lowly as we are, we each can say as Mary did; "For He who is mighty has done great things for me, and holy is His name" (Lk 1:49). (See Appendix II for a chronological presentation, in litany form, of the events and experiences Mary lived as the first Christian believer.)

The Bold Journey of Hope

Reflecting upon the Christian life, particularly in the current turbulent age in which we live, we might paraphrase an old adage by saying that, for the Christian: all roads lead to Bethlehem. With Unborn Jesus and His parents we are traveling that meandering prophetic road to the place of birth of God's child and of every child. Will the unborn child make it to Bethlehem to be counted among the living or will the unborn child be killed along the way? We must try to help and protect the unborn child on this journey (and assist the parents as necessary) and see in him or her a living image of Unborn Jesus.

CHAPTER EIGHT ENDNOTES

1. Pope John Paul II, *Apostolic Exhortation Guardian of the Redeemer,* trans. Vatican (Boston: St. Paul Books & Media, 1989), # 9, 16-17.
2. H. W. van der Vaart Smit, *Born In Bethlehem,* trans. Thomas R. Milligan (Baltimore, MD: Helicon Press, Inc., 1963), 17-21.
3. In a way the Bethlehem census can be linked to every human census. But in a most remarkable way it was prefigured – inversely – by the "census" count conducted by God at Sodom and Gomorrah (which cities represented worldliness in every age; Gen 18:1-19:28). Abraham proposed that the righteous souls be counted, hoping that the cities would be spared. But only Lot was found to be righteous – not enough to save them. In Bethlehem, Caesar would count the baby Jesus failing to understand what he was counting – the Savior who could save us all from eternal destruction. The Sodom and Gomorrah event underscores the fruitless pursuits of misguided souls leading to death. Whereas the Bethlehem event points to the fruit of Mary's womb, Jesus who brings us Eternal Life. Both episodes end in frantic flights from danger. The two angels seize Lot (and family), Joseph and Mary seize the baby Jesus, and flee.
4. St. Thomas Aquinas, O.P.,Summa Theologica, I, Question 35, Art. 7.
5. Raphael Brown, ed., *The Life of Mary As Seen by the Mystics* (Rockford, IL: Tan Books and Publishers, Inc., 1951), 101.
6. Mother St. Paul, *Ortus Christi* (London: Longmans, Green And Co. Ltd., 1921), 106-107.
7. Rev.Frederick W. Faber, C.O., D.D., *Bethlehem* (Baltimore, MD: John Murphy & Co.), 95.
8. Mother St. Paul, *Ortus Christi,* op. cit., pp.97-98.
9. St. Bede, O.S.B., *Super Lucam.* ii.4,5.
10. One of St. Paul's great quotes about the attitude adopted by Jesus when He came into the world is Phil 2:5-7, which states in part, that Christ Jesus "emptied himself, taking the form of a servant…". This was quoted and discussed in chapter one. In the Knox translation of the New Testament the last phrase is translated as; "took the nature of a slave".
11. Billy Graham, *Peace With God* (Nashville, TN: Thomas Nelson, Inc., 1984), 114.
12. John Donne, Holy Sonnet, Annunciation.
13. St. Alphonsus de Liguori, C.S.S.R.,*The Incarnation, Birth and Infancy of Jesus Christ* (Brooklyn, NY: Redemptorist Fathers, 1927), 227-228.
14. Dear reader, when I began this book in the late 1980's and first came across the previous quote by Alphonsus de Liguori, I felt it was too neg-

ative to include in this book. But as the years passed, I became convinced that when Jesus was in the womb for nine months it was, in a mystical sense, a time of solidarity with all unborn infants who are deliberately killed by abortion. God knew that in our own misguided time, unborn babies would be sacrificed before they could be born and Unborn Jesus wanted in some way to share their cross. So, I decided that instead of excluding the foregoing quote from this book, I should definitely include it.

15. T. S. Eliot, *Four Quartets* (London: Faber And Faber, 1972), 38.
16. Before Mary and Joseph fled the Bethlehem/Jerusalem region with newborn Jesus to head towards Egypt, Mary had been repeatedly tutored by God, directly and indirectly; through God's angels and other faithful Israelites inspired by the Holy Spirit. In every instance she was either directly involved as a participant or as a witness, or the event was re-told directly to her by the one(s) who experienced it. Angels instructed Zechariah (Lk 1:5-25), Mary (Lk 1:26-38), Joseph (Mt 1:20, 2:13, 19, 22), the Bethlehem shepherds (Lk 2:8-20). The Holy Spirit inspired unborn baby John (Lk 1:41), Elizabeth (Lk 1:41-45), Mary (Lk 1:46-55), Zechariah (Lk 1:64-79), the wise men from the East (Mt 2:2, 11-12), Simeon (Lk 2:25-35) and the prophetess Anna (Lk 2:36-38).
17. David S. Yeago, "The Presence of Mary in the Mystery of the Church", *Mary Mother of God*, ed. Carl E. Braaten and Robert W. Jenson, (Grand Rapids, Michigan: William B. Eerdmans Publishing Company, 2004), 66-67, 69.

9

The Great Nativity

And while they were there, the time came for her to be delivered. And she gave birth to her first-born son and wrapped him in swaddling cloths, and laid him in a manger, because there was no place for them in the inn.

Luke 2:6-7

It is now time to consider the last event in the life of Christ while He is still in that hidden unborn state: His being born. For until He is born, He remains yet unborn. Before being born He is still unseen, unheard, untouched and unknown: Unborn Jesus.

Billions of words have been written and spoken about the birth of Jesus Christ. So instead, let us here consider the unborn Christ immediately prior to and even during the birth process, rather than the familiar post-birth scene.

First of all it must be stated that every baby about to be born is physiologically poised or primed for the process and moment. The baby is agitated and anxious as two physiologies push and play against each other anticipating their impending separation. Unborn Jesus would have felt similar human desires as well as deep divine desires. He was; "...waiting for the moment to come when He can take the next step in His earthly journey, waiting with His Mother whose intense desire is only second to His Own."[1]

If any words from the mouth of Christ might shed some light on the state of His being at this preborn point in time it would be those words uttered thirty or so years later in holy frustration; "I came to cast fire upon the earth; and would that it were already kindled! I have a baptism to be baptized with; and how I am constrained until it is accomplished!" (Lk 12:49-50) We see in these final hours before birth the last definitive stage of the astounding nine-month journey that each of us travels and that our Lord was here embracing for our sake. The preborn Christ Child is no longer content to be within His mother's body. His limbs, His nervous system, His hormones, His instincts, His Heart are all of one voice resounding within His innermost Self crying out to be born.

Now as He sets His course for the wide open world beyond His mother's body – a world where He will offer His own Body – He remains yet a baby. Once born He will cry and whimper, blink His eyes in disbelief, turn His tiny neck from side to side to see the world while clenching His little fists with fierce desire. His future lies outside the capsule of the womb. His life will never be the same again. Yet once outside He will still depend on this woman; the only Mother He ever knew.

Yes, the Savior wanted to be born, to see humans through His human eyes, to hear humans speak with His human ears, to touch and be touched, to smile and engender good will thereby. He, like every other preborn baby in the ninth month of gestation, wanted to be free of His space constraints, free of the womb. He wanted to be born!

No doubt Mary felt the same way. Standing, walking, bending over – even sleeping – all of these everyday actions were now accompanied by marked discomfort. Practical Joseph on the other hand, was probably still hoping to find a convenient time and place for the blessed event.

To See the Face of God and Live

For Mary there was welling up inside her now a simple desire; to see her son's face. She had known Him for nine months through a veil. Now she imagined herself within hours looking into her baby's face and holding Him against her; His Heart pressed against her own heart. Caryll Houselander wrote of these maternal longings: "Yet she must have longed to hold Him between her hands and to look into His human face and to see in it, in the face of God, a family likeness to herself!"[2] This longing was not egotistical but was a very young mother's heart reaching out to the distant child invisible to her yet sending her secret messages with every outward kick and poke. Her young heart was straining, almost to breaking, to behold the One Who loved her most, Who needed her most. Father Faber expounds upon her experience more fully in his book entitled *Bethlehem:*

> Now Mary's Expectation was full of God, and therefore it was joyous. It had two intensities of joy in it: the intensity of created holiness thirsting for the sight of God; and the intensity of an earthly mother's desire – natural, simple, and human, but immensely sanctified – to see the Face of her Babe, whom she knew to be God as well. . .Mary yearned for that earthly beatific Vision, the Face of the Incarnate God. She had doubtless intellectual visions, as mystics call them, of the beauty of the Sacred Humanity, before that night at Bethlehem. But these would rather increase the burning of her desire, than be a satisfaction to it. . .[3]

One popular devotion in the Church is the devotion to our Lord's Holy Face; particularly the face of the crucified Jesus. If we try to imagine the origin of such a devotion we must acknowledge that it could not have originated anywhere else but in Mary's maternal heart sometime prior to the birth of her cherished Son; perhaps here in Bethlehem. For devotion is but tender love directed toward God, and before loving her crucified Lord she loved her Unborn Lord. And the desire to see His newborn face would, by love, precede that desire to contemplate the crucified one. "Hear, O Lord, when I cry aloud, be gracious to me and answer me! Thou hast said, Seek ye my face. My heart says to thee, Thy face, Lord, do I seek. Hide not thy face from me" (Ps 27:7-9).[4]

Years later that Son would say to His followers; "Blessed are the pure in heart, for they shall see God" (Mt 5:8). Mary and Joseph were pure in heart and would have their desire to see God, their Son, fulfilled upon meeting Him face to face at His birth.

"His own people received Him not" (Jn 1:11)

We can not know exactly how these final events of the Savior's birth unfolded, but we may reflect upon the rendition St. Alphonsus de Liguori gives of that night:

> Mary knew that the time of her delivery was come, and that it was here, and on that night, that the Incarnate Word willed to be born, and to manifest Himself to the world. She therefore told Joseph, and he hastened to procure some lodging in the houses of the towns-people, so as not to take his spouse to the inn to be delivered, as it was not a decent place for her to be in; besides which, it was then full of people.
>
> But he found not any one to listen to him; and very likely he was insulted, and called a fool by some of them, for taking his wife about at that time of night, and in such a crowd of people, when she was near her delivery; so that at last he was obliged, unless he would remain all night in the street, to take her to the public inn, where there were many other poor people lodging that night. He went there; but they were refused admittance even there, and they were told that there was no room for them... There was room for all, even for the lowest, but not for Jesus Christ.

At this point St. Alphonsus digresses, comparing the inn to the human heart and lamenting so many closed doors. We continue:

> These poor travelers, then seeing themselves repulsed on every side, leave the city to try and find some place of refuge without its walls. They walk on in the dark; they go round about and examine, till at last they see a grotto, which was cut out of stone in the mountain under the city. Barradas, Bede, and Brocardus say that the place where Jesus Christ was born was a rock that had been excavated under the walls of Bethlehem, divided off from the city, and like a cavern, and which served as a stable for cattle.[5]

In her book, *Footsteps of the Master*, Harriet Beecher Stowe refers to the census as "the last step in the humiliation of their nation" and then focuses on Mary and Joseph's plight as St. Alphonsus has just described:

> ....what a trial and humiliation it was to these children of a royal race to find themselves outcasts and homeless in the city of their fathers – in the very hour when home and its comfort were most needed... left to touch the very lowest descent of humiliation, out-casts from among men, glad to find a resting place with the beasts of the stall.[6]

If the census was a blatant expression of domination by the Roman Empire over its subject nations, and the Messiah and His parents are now rejected by His own people and kin, truly the humiliation was profound and complete – an appropriate finale to the nine months Unborn Jesus has spent in the womb of His mother.

And now we must pause to bring our modern hustle and bustle world to Bethlehem for a brief moment. There is one sentence that our Lord spoke towards the end of His ministry on earth that has to be applied to His unborn life. It is appropriate as we look back over His nine months experience within the womb to recall it now: "Truly, I say to you, as you did it to one of the least of these my brethren, you did it to me." (Mt 25:40)

How might we define today "the least of these my brethren"? There are many people who qualify as "the least" among us. They might be homeless, poor, sick, dying, weak, hungry, emotionally or mentally ill, disabled, rejected or neglected, needy young or elderly – even incarcerated. But certainly the unborn baby is the classic textbook case of a qualifying individual. For if we consider "least" in age, in size, in status, in wealth or power, in independence, in relationships or influence, in recognition or accomplishments, the unborn baby is always "least"!

This brings us to the shadow cast by the door of the inn at Bethlehem and the shadow cast by the innkeeper. An inn represents acceptance and welcoming hospitality and an innkeeper represents one whose responsibility it is to extend that attitude of consideration. But this unborn baby and His mother received no welcome, only deliberate rejection. Yet we find comfort in looking back at the five "Saints of the Incarnation" who did reach out to Unborn Jesus: Mary, unborn John, Elizabeth, Zechariah and Joseph (in this chronological order). But who will reach out to help unborn children today? Surely Unborn Jesus will guide us in answering this question.

The Perfect Setting for This Moment of Moments

The actions of Joseph and Mary in search of a place for the birth of the Son to occur seem to be a living and literal example of what our Lord would teach many years later, although it is not obvious to those of us who tend to script out in advance the answer to prayer that we want to receive: "Ask, and it will be given you; seek, and you will find; knock, and it will be opened to you" (Mt 7:7).

So it turned out that Jesus would be born not only in the "fullness of time" but in the ideal location; a cave used as a stable. How curious that they were of the House of David, and that this too was the City of David, yet they had no kinsfolk who would take them in. Perhaps other kinsfolk from distant locals had already filled up all of these households. Anyway, God wanted this Holy Family to go through this miraculous divine moment alone. And so they did. By this experience God has touched countless hearts through the centuries, and continues to do so even today.

We should appreciate all the circumstances of these last hours leading up to the Savior's birth, which are not accidental but purposely chosen by God as part of Revelation. For example, most appropriate was the "time of day" that Christ would be born; "the Light of the World" is born in the dark of night. Cardinal Cushing puts it this way:

> Christ was born in the midst of darkness. He was born deep in the night, so the tradition tells us. He was born in the gloom of a stable in the shadow of a darkened inn. But this physical darkness was in turn the symbol of a spiritual darkness embracing all the souls of men, overshadowed as these were by the corporate sins of the race.[7]

Nighttime and darkness are associated with various sins best committed when one cannot be seen so well (I Th 5:5, Rom 13:12). Why not then choose nighttime for the entrance of our Redeemer onto the stage of our humanity? "The people who walked in darkness have seen a great light; those who dwelt in a land of deep darkness, on them has light shined...For to us a child is born, to us a son is given..." (Is 9:2, 6).

The "place" where Christ will be born – in a cave – is also of great significance. G.K Chesterton notes that human history began with the famous "cave man" and then embellishes upon the Nativity observing that "God also was a Cave-Man":

> The second half of human history, which was like a new creation of the world, also begins in a cave....the rejoicings in the cavern were rejoicings in a fortress or an outlaw's den; properly understood it is not unduly flippant to say they were rejoicings in a dug-out. It is not only true that such a subterranean chamber was a hiding place from enemies; and that the enemies were already scouring the stony plain that lay above it like a sky. It is not only that the very horse-hoofs of

> Herod might in that sense have passed like thunder over the sunken head of Christ. It is also that there is in that image a true idea of an outpost, of a piercing through the rock and an entrance into an enemy territory. There is in this buried divinity an idea of undermining the world; of shaking the towers and palaces from below...[8]

Christ emerges from before time, secretly in a womb, within a cave, in the side of a mountain, in the dark of night. What could be more hidden than the interior of a womb in a cave in a mountain at night? Is this not creation's own hiding place? Yes, like a thief He will come in the night (Mt 24:43-44). And what better locale to unleash this Divine plot – the redemption of all humankind – than in this secluded out-of-the-way place? As the first Adam hid from God after sinning now this second Adam hides from the offspring of the first Adam as He sets out to redeem them all.

Recall how the prophet Elijah sought God in a cave on Mount Horeb (I Kings 19:9-13). God made Himself known to Elijah not in power and might, but rather in "a still small voice" which Elijah heard from within the cave. From there the Lord sent Elijah out on his mission. So, too, here in this Bethlehem cave, amidst the hushed prayers and whisperings of humans and angels alike, soon would come a little cry of newborn Divinity, muffled so as not to frighten any away – "a still small voice" – immediately to be sent out on the Mission of all missions.

How appropriate also – and not merely coincidental – that the birth place would turn out to be near the fields where the sheep grazed. It had been ordained that the last angelic "Annunciation of the Lord" would be to shepherds, who in their lowliness represent the very sheep they tended.[9] Had not the prophets spoken of the Messiah as one who would shepherd Israel? Now as infant Shepherd King he would come to them and like Abraham, Moses and King David, He would shepherd His sheep.

". . .the first-born of all creation" (Col 1:15)

Within hours the Son of God will be born. He will symbolically reach out to His creation to embrace it for the first time and to claim it as His own. Indeed, animal life, humans and angels will gather round Him at that moment to respond. Again and again St. Paul pointed to this mystery of relationship between the Lord Jesus Christ and His Creation. We are unable here to explore in detail this wondrous reality, but we can glance at it quickly as we move towards the glorious event, relying on Paul's teaching in two of his letters:

Col 1:16	for in him all things were created
Col 1:16	all things were created through him and for him
Col 1:17	he is before all things
Col 1:17	in him all things hold together
Col 1:20	through him to reconcile to himself all things
Col 1:18	that in everything he might be pre-eminent
Eph 1:10	a plan for the fullness of time, to unite all things in him
Eph 1:22	he has put all things under his feet
Eph 1:22	has made him the head over all things for the church
Col 1:15	He is the image of the invisible God, *the first-born of all creation*

When the Son of God came into the world, He already had a remarkable relationship to it. As the prologue to John's Gospel puts it: "He was in the beginning with God; all things were made through him, and without him was not anything made that was made." So we might say that all of creation was stamped with the royal seal of God's Son from the very start. With His Incarnation, the Son of God leaps across the great chasm of eternity to join us in our journey through history, one day at a time. To paraphrase St. Paul, we can say that "the Unborn Christ Child is pre-eminent in everything!" Then, after about 270 days, we come to this day when the Son of God will be recognized as the Son of Man; the first-born of all creation! He who was begotten by the Father before time is truly creation's first-born – not in time but in reality.

The specific focus of this Incarnation Mission is the salvation of humankind and their rehabilitation. Adam had a sort of temporary headship over creation, but he failed. God however had a long term plan in mind. Tertullian (155/160 A.D. - 240/250 A.D.) succinctly described the creation of Adam from the earth: "The shape that the slime of the earth was given was intended with a view to Christ, the future man."[10] In other words, Adam was "but a copy of the predestinated Humanity of Jesus".[11] We can conclude then that all of human development from the first cell stage onward was designed on the eternal plan for the Incarnate Christ. The unborn baby prototype was Unborn Jesus Himself.[12] St. Francis de Sales (1567-1622) explains it this way:

> ...if someone intends to build a house or a palace he must first consider whether it is to be a lodging for a vine dresser or a peasant or if it is for a lord, since obviously he would use entirely different plans depending on the rank of the person who is to live there. Now the Eternal Father did just that when he built this world. He intended to create it for the Incarnation of His Son, the Eternal Word. The end or goal of His work was thus its beginning, for Divine Wisdom had foreseen from all eternity that His Word would assume our nature in coming to earth.[13]

So the model for the first Adam (and every human being thereafter) sprang from the Eternal and Infinite Mind of God as He contemplated the Second Adam; the Eternal Adam. So perhaps for discussion's sake we can paraphrase a statement Jesus made one day about Abraham (Jn 8:58): "Truly, truly, I say to you, before 'Adam' was, I am." And when He is born, He will be the first-born of all creation, and He will be the Head of all things – just as the three wise men from the East suspected.

And now, as God is about to be born among the children of Adam and Eve, and history's underpinnings are about to be turned upside down, might be a good time to pause and take one last look backwards at the past nine months of this one-of-a-kind redemptive pregnancy.

Nine Months Preparation and the Forming of His Sacred Humanity

The body of Jesus has been growing and developing now for almost nine months. He is living the mystery of the Incarnation in secret but soon will live it in the light of day. He is fully God and fully man. His life is the turning point of human history, beginning at the one cell stage of His human life. Cardinal Schonborn enlightens us on a critical aspect of the Incarnation:

> Here Christ's conception through the Spirit acquires its full range of application: here is one man whose existence is entirely new, right from its root. In the midst of a world where anything new simply replaces something old, only to become old in its turn, there is now a new humanity, a human life which does not, at its conception, have the germ of death in it, but comes forth entirely out of God's newness.[14]

The sacred humanity of Jesus is distinctly new and fresh. Ronald Knox says that through the Incarnation God "had infected the human race, as it were, with His Divinity".[15] For months the body and life of Unborn Jesus has been forming, preparing for birth and then life after birth. (Once born, He will be preparing for death and then life after death.) The exciting part is that Jesus Christ has a permanent effect upon human destiny. His life will not get old and need to be replaced with something new again. No, His abundant life remains new and accessible for ever. And from the newness of Christ comes a New Creation for us all.

These months of growth and development within His mother's womb have been exhilarating and full of promise even if only a handful of people knew about it. For all has been going according to God's Plan. The body of Unborn Jesus was being formed and prepared for years of daily living and work, for public ministry, then ultimately for crucifixion, resurrection and eternity.

Consider the crucifixion in this light. The blood which will be shed in this sacrifice began to course through His body about eight months before His birth and would continue to run freely until that final offering.[16] Likewise, every physical feature of our Lord's body, while forming in the womb, took on its own predestined sacrificial character, a character that would be eternally stamped upon it during His Passion and death.

Various Psalms and prophetic books of the Old Testament described the passion of the Christ. One of the most famous of the "Passion Psalms" is psalm 22 which begins "My God, my God, why hast thou forsaken me?" Yet, even here we find a reference to Mary's womb where the Messiah was sheltered before birth. It is the Messiah, Jesus, who speaks to His Father: "Yet thou art he who took me from the womb; thou didst keep me safe upon my mother's breasts" (Ps 22.9). Perhaps the Messiah is here recognizing that even when He was still a baby – unborn, then newborn – He was being formed for the most dreadful of missions.

The Passion and death flower into the glory of the Resurrection! The Resurrection is the true fulfillment of the Incarnation.[17] Both events – within womb and tomb – marking the beginning and the ending of our Lord's ordinary earthly life among us, are accomplished by the power of God in complete and holy secrecy. The forming of the body of Unborn Jesus in the womb anticipated its later glorification within and beyond the tomb. Hence, the Incarnation of Jesus Christ was predestined to continue into eternity. That first cell of His body was the first cell of His new humanity, the first cell of His eternal body.

Similarly, for every baby the nine months within the womb is a sacred period of formation, a holy time of preparation with a personal providential plan in mind. The complete person, body and soul, is created by God for a purpose that awaits discovery.

> *For thou didst form my inward parts,*
> *thou didst knit me together in my mother's womb.*
> *I praise thee, for thou art fearful and wonderful.*
> *Wonderful are thy works!*
> *Thou knowest me right well;*
> *my frame was not hidden from thee,*
> *when I was being made in secret,*
> *intricately wrought in the depths of the earth.*
> *Thy eyes beheld my unformed substance;*
> *in thy book were written, every one of them,*
> *the days that were formed for me,*
> *when as yet there was none of them.*
>
> Psalm 139:13-16

The first nine lines quoted from this psalm are quite clear in meaning but the last three are more ambiguous.[18] Here is a different translation of those last three lines: "In Your book all my days were recorded, even those which were purposed before they had come into being."[19] In other words, even from those first days in the womb, God has a positive purpose and plan, not only for Unborn Jesus, but for every unborn child.

The Mystery of the Great Nativity

We have looked backward through nine months of formative development and forward to adult and eternal consequences of Christ's special preparation period within the womb. Now finally, we consider the impending birth. Given the background of Mary and Joseph (not to mention the messianic nature of the event) the experience within the cave must have been one of intense prayer – both silent and vocal. We are reminded at this intimate moment of human history, when the lives of Jesus, Mary and Joseph are undergoing such a blessed upheaval, of the teaching: "For where two or three are gathered in my name, there am I in the midst of them" (Mt 18:20). Literally all the words and deeds of that night were performed by the family – huddled in the cave – uniquely for the preborn baby Jesus and done in His Name.

Prayerfully then the event unfolds. The tenor of the prayer of Mary and Joseph must have been thanksgiving and praise and their mood one of anticipation, for they realized they were living and witnessing the immediate fulfillment of numerous messianic prophecies.

The final precious hours before the birth are charged with the intensity of divine love flowing through frail human channels. Joseph, anxious for his weary wife and the baby Jesus. Mary intent on the imminent birth and concerned for the comfort of her little one. Ready or not, the Messiah was coming.

"The Light of the World"
"The Word Made Flesh"
"The Son of God"
"Emmanuel"
"Jesus"

His birth, like His conception, was Divine mystery. During the present era, and in fact through the centuries, not a great deal has been said about the actual physiological moment and manner of His birth. The Gospels do not give details of the actual birth event. However, in the last chapter of the Book of Isaiah there are two verses which seem to apply to the birth of Jesus: "Before she was in labor she gave birth; before her pain came upon her she was delivered of a son. Who has heard such a thing? Who has seen such things?" (Isa 66:7-8)

For several reasons these prophetic verses are of great interest. Like other messianic verses, they are direct and to the point. Notice, however, that in a sense we have here the undoing of Eve's curse. That is the key to understanding these verses. ("I will greatly multiply your pain in childbearing; in pain you shall bring forth children...." Gen 3:16). Before God spoke this curse to Eve, He had promised the coming of the Messiah (See Gen 3:15). So the first promise of the Messiah was linked with the curse in childbearing. At any rate, Isaiah describes here the laborless and painless birth of a son. It seems that we have come full circle now, from the original creation of humanity and God's curse upon Eve for her grievous disobedience, to the New Creation in Christ Who is born through Mary's exemplary obedience and whose birth is exempt from Eve's legacy. It does sound miraculous, doesn't it? But in other respects was it "natural"? [20] Obviously we are dealing with a supreme mystery here. Some fathers of the Church did venture into this discussion. In his Letter to Volusian, St. Augustine touched briefly upon it: "That same power which afterwards brought the body of the young man (Jesus) through closed doors, brought the body of the infant forth from the inviolate virginal womb of the Mother. If you seek out the reason for this it will no longer be marvelous. If you demand a comparable example it will no longer be unique."[21]

There are others too, such as Pope St. Gregory (I) the Great, who have offered insights.[22] Nonetheless, exact details of the birth as experienced by Jesus and His mother are not revealed in scripture, and there is no reason why they should have been. Some beautiful qualities of our faith concern alternating layers of historical fact-upon-fact and spiritual mystery-upon-mystery. The actual birth of Jesus is like Heaven's sunrise. He comes from eternity, beyond the mystery of a timeless dark night via the transfigured rays of earth's daylight, eternally begotten of the Father and now temporally born of Mary, from Love's omnipotent source to be gentle Love's sign: "a babe wrapped in swaddling cloths" (Lk 2:12).

And so the nine-month hidden journey came to an end. What began miraculously in Heaven and northern Israel drew to a momentous conclusion in a cave in southern Israel. Heralded by angels at both outset and finale, yet quietly contrived and brought to completion.

This then was the first phase of the Incarnation of the Son of God! The most hidden and preliminary stage of the Incarnation Mission. With His birth would begin a new time of encountering the human community with His Grace and Truth. Looking back we see the stark impact He has already had on each life He has visited; there is the clear before-and-after of His Presence (B.C./A.D.). Virtually three generations were directly affected and exposed to this new Christ-centered way of living: unborn baby John, Mary and Joseph, and the elderly couple Elizabeth and Zechariah.

Having followed Him now from Nazareth to Bethlehem, we can recognize His "calling card", the trademark of Unborn Jesus. Messianic Joy! "In thy presence there is fullness of joy" (Ps 16:11). The Messiah's life from conception onward is punctuated with joy! As real as His own heartbeat, His joy pulsated through these initial unborn months. We witnessed this heavenly species of joy with the inspired leap "for joy" of unborn John in his mother's womb (Lk 1:44), in the prophetic canticle of Mary – "my spirit rejoices in God my Savior" (Lk 1:47) – and again in the angelic salutation to the shepherds; "...I bring you good news of a great joy..." (Lk 2:10).

Yet, through this nine-month period Unborn Jesus and His mother lived in three different homes, had journeyed the countryside on three occasions and now found themselves homeless, like animals living in a cave devoid of human comforts. Where was His real home? "Foxes have holes, and birds of the air have nests; but the Son of man has nowhere to lay his head" (Mt 8:20). The womb of His mother had been a true home for Him, but it was merely a temporary home, a sign of a truer home still.

Mary's heart would remain for Him, a permanent home. She had welcomed Him into her life with open arms. She gave to Him all she had. She carried Him simultaneously in heart and womb...later in her heart and arms...always in her heart!

CHAPTER NINE ENDNOTES

1. Mother St. Paul, *Ortus Christi* (London: Longmans, Green And Co. Ltd., 1921), 128.
2. Caryll Houselander, *The Reed of God* (Westminster, MD: Christian Classics, Inc., 1990), 41.
3. Rev. Frederick W. Faber, C.O., D.D., *Bethlehem* (Baltimore, MD: John Murphy & Co.), 89-91.
4. Also see Ps 11:7 and Num 6:24-26.
5. St. Alphonsus de Liguori, C.S.S.R.,*The Incarnation, Birth and Infancy of Jesus Christ* (Brooklyn, NY: Redemptorist Fathers, 1927), 142-143.
6. Harriet Beecher Stowe, *Footsteps of the Master* (New York: J. B. Ford & Co., 1877), 56.
7. Richard Cardinal Cushing, *Christ in Bethlehem, Christ in the Eucharist* (Boston: St. Paul Editions), 81.
8. G. K. Chesterton, *The Everlasting Man* (New York: Dodd, Mead & Company, 1925), 201,217-218.
9. The angelic Annunciation of the Lord to Mary occurred immediately before the pregnancy, the angelic Annunciation of the Lord to Joseph occurred midway during the pregnancy and the last angelic Annunciation of the Lord to the shepherds occurred immediately after the pregnancy.
10. Tertullian, *De Carnis Resurrectione.*
11. Rev. Frederick W. Faber, C.O., D.D., *The Blessed Sacrament* (Baltimore, MD: John Murphy Company, circa 1855), 445.
12. Alan Keenan, O.F.M., *Neuroses and Sacraments* (London: Sheed and Ward, 1950), 64-67.
13. Rev. Lewis S. Fiorelli, O.S.F.S., ed., *The Sermons of St. Francis de Sales for Advent and Christmas,* trans. Nuns of the Visitation (Rockford, IL: Tan Books and Publishers, Inc., 1987), 83.
14. Cardinal Christoph von Schonborn, O.P. *The Mystery of the Incarnation,* trans. Graham Harrison (San Francisco: Ignatius Press, 1992), 48.
15. Rev. Ronald A. Knox, *The Hidden Stream* (London: Burns Oates, 1952), 12.
16. "By day 22, a primitive heart, shaped as a tube in a loop, begins to beat. Thus, very primitive blood cells start to circulate through forming minute blood vessels." Stuart Campbell, M.D., *Watch Me Grow* (New York: St. Martin's Griffin, 2004), 14.
17. *Catechism of the Catholic Church,* trans. United States Catholic Conference (Citta del Vaticano: Libreria Editrice Vaticana, 1994), 170 (#653).

18. Verse 13 is also of interest. The expression "knit me together" is describing a planned growth process in which God is actively involved. But St. Paul uses the same terminology in two letters describing the early growth process of the Church (Eph 4:15-16 and Col 4:19). Paul would have known this Psalm well, perhaps even by heart. It is quite possible that he specifically chose this terminology because he had an image of an embryonic (Church) Body still in the early formative stages in mind.
19. *The Bible in Basic English*, Cambridge Univ. Press and E.P. Dutton and Company.
20. For a more detailed summary of historical teachings and viewpoints on this topic see: Dr. Ludwig Ott, *Fundamentals of Catholic Dogma*, trans. Patrick Lynch, Ph.D. (Rockford, Il: Tan Books and Publishers, Inc., 1974), 205-206 (Book Three, Part 3, Chp. 2, #5).
21. William A. Jurgens, *The Faith of the Early Fathers*, Vol. 3 (Collegeville, MN: The Liturgical Press, 1979), 6. As briefly noted earlier in this chapter, the risen Body of Jesus Christ is the same Body as was crucified but possesses new properties as a glorious and transfigured Body. At birth, His is a natural physical Body, not a glorious transfigured one. Nonetheless, throughout His life Jesus repeatedly demonstrated supernatural Divine powers over nature, physical matter and otherwise. Was His birth natural or supernatural as to the physiological process? Did the Holy Spirit intervene miraculously in the process? The answers seem shrouded in mystery.
22. IBID., 323.

EPILOGUE
ON PRAYING TO UNBORN JESUS

How do you picture Jesus when you pray to Him? Do you focus on a particular attribute or aspect of His being or personality as you relate to Him and pray to Him? St. John the evangelist got a real surprise one Sunday on the island of Patmos when he had his famous vision, recorded for all time in the Book of Revelation. This is how John described Jesus: "...His head and His hair were white as white wool, white as snow; His eyes were like a flame of fire, His feet were like burnished bronze....and His face was like the sun shining in full strength"(Rev 1:14-16).

We don't normally think of Jesus as having white hair or eyes like flaming fire. John later saw Jesus again during this same vision, but this time He was a Lamb being worshipped by thousands (Rev 5:5-13). In fact, just to assure myself that I had not misunderstood, I consulted many different Biblical Commentaries and they all confirmed that the white haired Person and the Lamb were indeed Christ the Lord. Somehow I get the impression that God's eternal heavenly perspective is a lot different from ours and that He is, or will be, present to us in extraordinary ways – a divinely creative presence which certainly will not be limited by our little minds.

Which brings us to Unborn Jesus. Could Jesus, who presents Himself to the beloved disciple as an ancient-looking white haired person "like a son of man", also present Himself to us as He once historically appeared on earth – say as an unborn baby, or a newborn, or a young boy of twelve years? Of course He could.

It would be futile to try and guess God's age in eternity. If you figure Jesus as "thirty something", think again. One New Testament writer proclaims that: "Jesus Christ is the same yesterday and today and for ever" (Heb 13:8). But what exactly does that mean in heaven, in eternity? The author C. S. Lewis has a short chapter in his book *Mere Christianity* devoted to the topic of God's eternal nature. He comments:

> God is not hurried along in the Time-stream of this universe any more than an author is hurried along in the imaginary time of his own novel. . . .If you picture Time as a straight line along which we have to travel, then you must picture God as the whole page on which the line is drawn. . . .But God, I believe, does not live in a Time-series at all. . . .You can not fit Christ's earthly life in Palestine into any time-relations with His Life as God beyond all space and time. . . .This human life in God is from our point of view a particular period in the history of the world (from the year A.D. one till the Crucifixion). We therefore imagine it is also a period in the history of God's own existence. But God has no history.[1]

While "God has no history", He most certainly has a life. True, He is no longer an unborn baby on earth, but He was, and even now is the Lord of all unborn babies and one with them. He was an adolescent and is one with adolescents today as their Lord too. People at every stage of life and in any situation whatsoever are His and He is their Lord now. Adults are mistaken if they believe that the only way to picture Jesus is as a "thirty something" adult.

People are different – that is how God planned it. Jesus is our Lord and Redeemer, but some will intensely focus on additional aspects of His person: teacher, healer, advocate, suffering servant, victor and so on. Similarly, there are various titles and names by which we are free to address Jesus both in prayer and intellectually: Word of God, Son of Man, Prince of Peace, Lamb of God, Good Shepherd, Christ the King and countless others. God does not want to limit us in any legitimate positive images and concepts that we develop concerning our Savior. In fact, I think God wants to encourage us to discover new and helpful insights about Christ our Lord.

Let's consider specifically one type of prayer – praise – and reflect on the diversity of praise that can be given to God. To help us in this exercise, picture a vast exquisite botanical garden surrounded by a multiplicity of specialized gardens representing the native plant life of all the geographical territories of the world. All of these types and variations of flowers and trees – hundreds of thousands of them – can symbolize the countless varied ways in which Christians can legitimately praise God.

Throughout the Bible – particularly in the Psalms – we find all kinds of examples of humans and creation praising God. It is as if God inspires within His people a multi-faceted approach to praise and then takes delight in it. Psalm 148 for example exhorts all manner of created things to praise God and concludes focusing particularly on praising "the name of the Lord, for his name alone is exalted". Surely it is also fitting that we praise the name and Person of Unborn Jesus as well!

If St. John can turn to Jesus as an ancient "son of man" in the first chapter of Revelation and worship Him and pray to Him as such, we can also turn to Him in simple childlike fashion as Unborn Jesus and pray to Him in like manner. "Fear not, I am the first and the last, and the living one; I died, and behold I am alive for ever more..." (Rev 1:17-18) Especially, we can petition Unborn Jesus on behalf of those unborn brothers and sisters of ours whose lives may be endangered by abortion. Surely Unborn Jesus had – and has – a special place in His most tiny hidden heart for today's vulnerable unborn children.

Indeed, Jesus Christ initiated His redemptive mission on earth from the womb, with a tender baby's heart. And how might we honor Him in those earliest moments, weeks and months? In a spirit of thanksgiving we can present Him with titles of honor and reverence: Unborn Christ Child, Unborn Lord, Unborn King, Unborn Savior, Unborn Son of God, Unborn Jesus of Nazareth, Unborn Guest (to unborn John the Baptist for example, and later in Bethlehem, as He figuratively knocks on the door at the inn), and so on.

In his book *A Retreat For Lay People*, Ronald Knox suggests that in the mystery of heavenly existence we will not only be privileged to see Christ in His glory, but also to see Him in His humanity, and not just one static picture of His humanity but perhaps all of His humanity in its various stages and events.

> But it seems difficult to believe that we shall have no sight, in heaven, of what Bethlehem was; and if of Bethlehem, why not of Calvary? I like to think, at least, that the three chaplets of the rosary will not shew any longer, in heaven, as three separate strands of experience, but somehow as a single tapestry. That seeing them both in their glory, we shall only have to bend sideways, as it were, to catch sight of

> the eternal truth in a different light; to see a Child resting in his Mother's arms; to see, though it were only one moment of eternity, our Lord's wounds still bleeding, and our Lady's tears.[2]

This perspective on heaven is childlike and wrestles with how humans might "experience" and relate to Jesus and mysteries of salvation "history" in Heaven. Let us not be too quick to construct limitations on how God might present Himself to us in eternity. Likewise let us enjoy our Christian freedom in approaching Jesus now, today, in prayer as the Spirit leads.

I believe that God wants to hear humanity cry out with prayers and praise to Unborn Jesus, that it pleases God to hear this special prayer in this sad time when the personhood and dignity of unborn babies is literally being mocked and their right to life being despised and disputed. I believe that God is encouraging us to see Him in His infancy and unborn state and to honor Him in that unborn state, and that as a direct result of honoring Him we will consequently honor all unborn children who are created in His image and likeness.

Nine Reasons to Honor Unborn Jesus

When we honor, pray to, and have a devotion to Unborn Jesus, we are:

1. Praising and glorifying God in a way that is pleasing to Him
2. Thanking God for the gift of the Incarnation – and our own redemption
3. Learning more about Jesus and His Incarnation Mission
4. Participating in the Church's tradition of honoring the Christ Child
5. Expanding our prayer life with the power of simple childlike prayer
6. Witnessing to the Gospel of Life in a beautiful and personal way
7. Honoring all unborn children who are like Unborn Jesus in many ways
8. Opening our hearts to pray for all unborn children at risk
9. Acknowledging our Lord's identification and solidarity with unborn babies – especially those who have died or are threatened by abortion

EPILOGUE ENDNOTES

1. C.S. Lewis, *Mere Christianity* (New York: Simon & Shuster, 1996), 147-149.
2. Rev. Ronald Knox, *A Retreat for Lay People* (Harrison, N.Y.: Roman Catholic Books, 1954), 170.

Appendix I
Identity and Personhood of the Incarnate Son of God

Just as today factions within society challenge and question the personhood and identity of unborn children, so too in the early centuries of Christianity the personhood and identity of Jesus Christ was repeatedly called into question. How many persons, natures, wills, intellects, bodies, souls are there in the God-man Jesus Christ? To tackle these questions the Church had to formalize new concepts which could adequately explain the realities embedded within this fundamental mystery of faith. Terms such as Trinity, Incarnation, Hypostatic Union and others – which do not appear in Sacred Scripture – were relied upon to clarify the Christian faith. The Council of Chalcedon in 451 A.D., for example, said of Jesus Christ:

> We declare that in his divinity he was begotten of the Father before time, and in his humanity he was begotten in this last age of Mary the Virgin, the Mother of God, for us and for our salvation.
>
> We declare that the one selfsame Christ, only-begotten Son and Lord, must be acknowledged in two natures without any commingling or change or division or separation; that the distinction between the natures is in no way removed by their union but rather that the specific character of each nature is preserved and they are united in one person and one hypostasis.

In the above complex formulation the term "*hypostasis*" is used. John Hardon, S.J. explains that to be united hypostatically "means that the two natures in Christ are united *personally,* in such a way that while the source *from* which the union was effected was two distinct natures, which remained essentially unchanged, the being in which the union was completed was one individual (in Greek, *hypostasis*), which individual was divine."[1] (Note: An excellent quick source for more insight on this topic is the *Catechism of the Catholic Church*, for example #464.)

It is important to recognize the fact that Jesus Christ is *one* person only, and that the union of the two natures occurs *in* the person of the Son of God. We analyze this in terms of the unique person-to-nature relationship enjoyed by Jesus Christ. One uncreated person (divine) assumed one created body and soul (human), yet there are two natures; that is, two intellects (divine and human) and two wills (divine and human). The unique make-up of this one God-man is an infinite mystery. And this is true from the first moment Christ is conceived by the power of the Holy Spirit, through the nine months in the womb, and ever after.

Now, as we mull over this personhood of Jesus, we may well wonder what He knew as to His divine intellect and His human intellect, and at what stages in His development. Simplistically, we can say that He had two kinds of knowledge: divine (infinite) knowledge, and human knowledge (three types of human knowledge: beatific knowledge, infused knowledge, and acquired – that is, experiential – knowledge). From the first moment of His conception He enjoyed the same divine knowledge which He had enjoyed from all eternity, but He also had human beatific and infused knowledge as well.

Perhaps a child-like image might help us to picture the unusual concept of the hypostatic union which exists in the Person of Jesus. The brilliant twentieth century philosopher Jacques Maritain came up with a simple fairy-tale-like visual image to depict the operations that might be occurring simultaneously in two different natures within one and the same person:

> Let us imagine an enormous giant, so tall that his head is higher than the layer of clouds from which falls an abundant rain on the earth. He climbs a mountain, whose summit is also higher than this layer of clouds; there he will be able to stretch himself out and sleep in the azure. Soaked by the rain, his body, while waiting, strides along under the clouds, from which it will emerge completely only at the end. But from the beginning his head is already in the azure and it enjoys it fully.[2]

This is a quaint physical image which might help us appreciate how Jesus could function volitionally and intellectually. It seems to paint two different worlds layered above and below the clouds, but they are part of one whole reality. If the giant sat down he would be seeing one "world", but if he stands up he sees the other and experiences them both simultaneously. Even if he chooses to sit, he knows full well what is above the clouds and can access that "world" in mere seconds. Admittedly, this limited image cannot and does not do justice to the glorious mystery of the Incarnation of the Son of God.

We are considering here a divine person in utero. Multiple mysteries engage us as we strive to glimpse divine love and life incarnate in Unborn Jesus Christ. We can ask ourselves, "When Jesus acts, does He act through His divine nature, His human nature or both?" Many theories abound which try to answer this question, but perhaps a concise and straightforward approach, as taken by Karl Adam is the most useful one:

> Scholasticism has come to distinguish three kinds of activity in Christ. Firstly, the purely divine acts. These are the actions brought about by the Logos before its incarnation – for example, the creation. They were wrought exclusively by the divine nature as the *principium quo.* In distinction to these, there are the purely human acts. These are the actions which, by their very character, belong exclusively to Jesus' human nature, actions like seeing, weeping, suffering, and so on. . . .The third kind of activity in Christ consists of those actions which are in fact accomplished by the Logos through the divine nature, but in such a way that in doing so he makes use of his human nature as an instrument.[3]

Throughout this book we often consider acts of Unborn Jesus Christ which would fall under this third categorization, acts accomplished by the Divine Logos while utilizing His human nature – extraordinary acts which will nonetheless harmonize with His human nature, in a sense, complementing that nature.

APPENDIX I ENDNOTES

1. Rev. John Hardon, S.J., *The Catholic Catechism* (Garden City, N.Y.: Doubleday & Company, Inc., 1975), 136.
2. Jacques Maritain, *On the Grace and Humanity of Jesus,* trans. Joseph W. Evans (New York: Herder and Herder, 1969), 69.
3. Karl Adam, *The Christ of Faith,* trans. Joyce Crick (New York: The New American Library of World Literature, Inc., 1957), 246.

Appendix II
Prayers Honoring the Incarnation of Jesus Christ

LITANY OF THE UNBORN CHRIST CHILD

Our Father, Author of Life,
Thank You for the gift of life.

Word of God, through Whom all things were made,
Thank You for the gift of life.

Holy Spirit, hovering over the waters of Creation,
Thank You for the gift of life.

Jesus, Your coming was announced by an angel,

* BLESS THE UNBORN AND THEIR PARENTS.

Jesus, conceived in love by God's Spirit and the Virgin Mary,*
Jesus, beloved son of a humble carpenter,*
Jesus, source of immeasurable joy for Mary and Joseph,*
Jesus, the aging Elizabeth rejoiced in Your presence,*
Jesus, You filled the unborn Baptist with gladness,*
Jesus, Mary's soul mirrors this gift of Divinity,*
Jesus, because of You all generations call Mary blessed,*
Jesus, one month in the womb and Your tiny heart beat for love,*
Jesus, another month passed and Your mouth and hands were wonderfully formed,*
Jesus, that mouth would tell the glory of God,*
Jesus, those hands were fashioned to be pierced for love,*
Jesus, before birth You rested near Your mother's faithful heart,*
Jesus, grateful to those who assisted Your mother during pregnancy,*

Jesus, teaching us; whatever we do to the least of Your brothers and sisters, we do to You,*
Jesus, Your birth was a joyful revelation to humanity,*
Jesus, days after that nativity, a fearful king planned to kill You,*
Jesus, countless infants were slaughtered in Your place,*

Lord, thank You for first coming among us as the Unborn Christ Child. Today, untold numbers of our tiny sisters and brothers have been abandoned by the world's leaders, by the traditional defenders of justice, by the healing professions and even by their own parents. But You are their Savior – You have not forgotten them. Savior, rescue and protect these little ones from the neglect and violence of an uncaring world.

Merciful Lord, Your tiny infant heart, which was later emptied on the cross, offers this world its only hope. Forgive us our sins against the unborn, against their parents and against all Your children. Lord, have mercy on us. Christ, have mercy on us. Lord, have mercy on us.

Prince of Peace, through Your healing Spirit, help us to lovingly accept every conceived child created in Your image and likeness, as a messenger of peace and goodwill towards all people. Amen.

LITANY IN HONOR OF MARY, THE FIRST CHRISTIAN

God Most High, we thank You for the merciful Incarnation of our Lord and Savior Jesus Christ.

God Most High, we honor You in the redemptive Incarnation of our Lord and Savior Jesus Christ.

God Most High, we praise You for the glorious Incarnation of our Lord and Savior Jesus Christ.

Our Lady of the Incarnation, pray for us.

Mary, chosen by God before the foundation of the world, — Eph 1:4/Gen 3:15

* PRAY FOR US WHO BELIEVE IN YOUR SON.

Mary, ever-virgin, chosen to be the Messiah's mother, * — Isa 7:14/Mt 1:22-23/Lk 1:26-27

Mary, clothed in humility and receptive to the will of God, * Lk 1:30,38,45,48,52

Mary, model of trust in motherhood, * Lk 1:29-31, 38

Mary, handmaid of the Lord, you conceived Christ Jesus by the Holy Spirit of God, * Lk 1:31, 35, 38

Mary, faithful Daughter of Zion, blessed are you for believing, * Zeph 3:16-20 /Lk 1:45-48

Mary, ever-faithful, you are the First Christian believer, * Lk 1:45-49

Mary, fervent disciple, you carry Unborn Jesus to His people, * Lk 1:39-40, 56

Mary, witness to the ministry of Messiah's prophet, * Lk 1:41-79

Mary, Ark of the New Covenant, you hold the Unborn Lord for nine prophetic months, * II Sam 6:9, 11/ Lk 1:43,45/ Rev 11:19-12.2

Mary, Bethlehem-bound to fulfill age-old prophecies, * Mt 2:3-6/Lk 2:4-7

Mary, in giving birth to Christ the Lord, you brought Joy to the world, * Lk 2:7, 10-11

Mary, babe-in-arms, you present the Savior to our world, * Lk 2:8-18/Mt 2:7-12

Mary, you devoutly carried the infant God into His Temple, * Lk 2:21-38

Mary, Messianic prophecies were revealed to you, * Lk 2:25-38

Mary, Protectress of our Savior, you sheltered Him from persecution, * Mt 2:13-23/ Rev 12:1-17

Mary, Mother of God, you nurtured and taught your child Jesus, * Mt 2:19-23/ Lk 2:39-41

Mary, you guided your Son to maturity in His religious observance, * Lk 2:41-52

Mary, at your signal Jesus Christ performed His first miracle-sign, *	Jn 2:3, 5, 11
Mary, you traveled with Jesus as He began His public ministry, *	Jn 2:12
Mary, faithful to the end, you witnessed your Son's cruel death, *	Jn 19:25-26/ Lk 2:34-35
Mary, after the crucifixion you were a mother to the beloved apostle John, *	Jn 19:26-27
Mary, you were the unique contemplative heart of the early Christian community, *	Act 1:12-15 (Lk 2:19,33,48,51)
Mary, at Pentecost, once again God's Spirit overshadowed you, *	Act 1:14-15, 2:1-4
Mary, Precursor of the Church and prophetically revealed in Heaven, *	Rev 12:1-17
Mary, you are Mother to Jesus and to His Body the Church, *	Jn 19:26-27/ Rev 12:17

Let Us Pray

O God, Most High, when You regarded the low estate of Your handmaiden Mary, she said: "He who is mighty has done great things for me, and holy is His name." Thank You Lord for choosing Mary as an integral instrument in the glorious Incarnation of Jesus Christ, our Savior. We also thank You for those "great things" You have done for Your Church and for each one of us personally. And Lord, as we strive daily to follow Jesus, may we remember all those who have gone before us faithfully blazing the trail of Jesus Christ. Amen.

ANGELUS OF PRAISE

Thank you God for the great and glorious Incarnation of our Lord and Savior Jesus Christ.

V. The angel of the Lord declared unto Mary.
R. And she conceived of the Holy Spirit.

Hail Mary, full of grace! The Lord is with thee, blessed art thou among women, and blessed is the fruit of thy womb, Jesus. Holy Mary, Mother of God, pray for us sinners, now and at the hour of our death.

All praise, glory, honor, thanksgiving and adoration are Yours O God Most High and most tiny, hidden heart of Unborn Jesus.

V. Behold the handmaid of the Lord.
R. Be it done unto me according to thy word.

Hail Mary......

All praise......

V. And the Word was made flesh.
R. And dwelt among us.

Hail Mary......

All praise......

Our Lady of the Incarnation, pray for us.
Mother of Hope, pray for us. Amen.

Note: The *Angelus* devotion recommended by Pope John XXII in the 14th century is a prayer for peace. It honors the Incarnation and promotes devotion to Mary. The practice developed of praying the *Angelus* in early morning, at midday and towards evening. Unfortunately, today the prayer is not frequently recited. The ***Angelus of Praise*** is a new modified format of the original *Angelus*, focusing more directly on Unborn Jesus, yet sharing the spiritual purpose of that ancient devotion.

APPENDIX III
THE "HAIL MARY" PRAYER

The well-known Catholic prayer – the Hail Mary – is a prayer which celebrates the Incarnation of Jesus Christ and focuses on that event and its implications for those of us who believe. The words of this scriptural and inspired prayer, are directed to Mary, who is the mother of Jesus and the first Christian. As we ask other Christians to pray for us, so too we can ask the first Christian, who has experienced the fullness of our Lord's Resurrection, to pray to her Son for us.

Over the centuries billions of words have been spoken and written about this prayer. Here we will take a different approach and consider it in relation to Unborn Jesus.

Hail Mary, full of grace
the Lord is with thee.
Blessed art thou among women
and blessed is the fruit
of thy womb
J
e
J e s u s
u
s.
Holy Mary,
Mother of God
pray for us sinners
now and at the hour of our death.
Amen.

The text of the prayer is presented above in a visual format so as to demonstrate that Unborn Jesus is at the core of this prayer and is its focus. (To further illustrate this point, we could also format the wording of the prayer in concentric circles, with the name Jesus at the center.) First of all, this prayer bears witness to the fact that we can not separate an unborn child from His mother. This prayer reflects on Mary during her pregnancy.

The first two sentences are from the Gospel of Luke. "Hail Mary, full of Grace, the Lord is with thee" (Lk 1:28). These are the words used by the archangel Gabriel to address Mary when he was announcing the Incarnation of Jesus. The announcement was immediately followed by her conception of Jesus.

The second sentence is spoken by Elizabeth, perhaps a week later, when pregnant Mary first arrives at the home of Elizabeth and Zechariah. Elizabeth is about six months pregnant with John the Baptist, and her unborn son leaps for joy within her upon the arrival of Mary and Unborn Jesus. Then Elizabeth is inspired by the Holy Spirit and cries out, "Blessed art thou among women and blessed is the fruit of thy womb!" (Lk 1:42). Note the scriptural exclamation mark ending these words. Now Elizabeth did not know the name of Mary's unborn son so her double blessing ends right there. And it is at this point where the Church has added the name of "Jesus" to these prophetic words of Elizabeth. (The archangel Gabriel had of course already announced the child's name.) So the prayer blesses Mary and then blesses Unborn Jesus. Elizabeth's greeting combines the two blessings just as Mary's body incorporates both individuals.

Still considering these words spoken by Gabriel and Elizabeth, we note that Gabriel is remarking on the disposition of Mary as being pleasing to God, while Elizabeth is blessing Mary for her relationship to the Lord, as mother. Whenever we pray it is important that we have a similar disposition to that of Mary and that we maintain a faithful relationship as well to her Son, our Savior.

When we pray "blessed is the fruit of thy womb, Jesus" we are specifically focusing upon Unborn Jesus. The words refer directly to that reality and we are repeating words spoken by Elizabeth at an historical point during Mary's pregnancy. So the heart of this prayer is one word: Jesus. Or rather, one Person: Jesus. But before dwelling at length upon this central aspect of the prayer, let us consider its concluding words.

The Church has added the following words "Holy Mary, Mother of God, pray for us sinners now and at the hour of our death." As we shall see these words are in keeping with the mother-child relationship that is key to this prayer. In the first part of the prayer we recall the Incarnation of Jesus while in the second part of the prayer we recall, albeit indirectly, His dying on the cross with His mother at His side praying for Him (Jn 19:25-27). So, at the conclusion of the prayer, we ask Mary in a child-like way, to be mother-like towards us "at the hour of our death" just as she was at the hour of our Lord's death.

In fact, in the same passage from St. John's Gospel Jesus entrusts "the disciple whom he loved" to His mother Mary. So it is logical for "disciples" who love Jesus to turn to His mother, and theirs, in the hour of need. While identifying Mary by her glorious vocation as Mother of God, the last sentence then asks her to pray for us "now". Just as Mary cared for her only Son all through His childhood, we implore her help for us children of God now in our lives.

The words of this prayer are assembled in such a way as to reflect the very image of the pregnant Mother Mary. Hidden within the midsection of this simple prayer is He who was hidden within the very womb of Mary His Mother: "Jesus". If we consider the prayer's components to be like a human figure, we see that the head and upper body of the prayer originate in Heaven, being angelic and inspired words. The midsection of the prayer is the hidden Unborn Jesus: "like treasure hidden in a field" or the "pearl of great value" (Mt 13:44-46). The lower body of the prayer consists of earthly intentions and desires as expressed by the Church. So the prayer mingles heavenly inspirations with earthly aspirations which coalesce around the God-man Jesus Christ Who is at the heart of this prayer.

Like the icons painted by Eastern Orthodox painters which always show the baby Jesus in Mary's embrace and Mary gracefully pointing to her son, so this prayer draws the one who prays to a secret center point: Jesus "the fruit" of Mary's womb. For even in nature we often find that the key reality is that which is hidden: the pearl buried within the oyster, the nut housed within the shell, the pebble from which concentric ripples are formed across the water.

Every time someone prays the "Hail Mary" prayer he or she is lifting up the hidden mystery of the Incarnation to be honored, in Spirit and in truth. While it is a prayer to the mother, both mother and Son are honored by the prayer. But from a more profound supernatural perspective we realize that "the fruit of (her) womb" is all in all, true God from true God, and is first in the order of Grace and Honor. Yet by the very nature of His Incarnation, in the womb, we see that Jesus desires in a most special manner to share the honor of His Person and Incarnation with His mother who collaborated uniquely in these mysteries.

We can say, then, that this prayer has a center point, and that is the name of "Jesus". It is this name which St. Paul says "is above every name" and at whose utterance "every knee should bow" (Phil 2:9-11). So when we pray this prayer, we are afforded an opportunity to show reverence to our Lord as we repeat His Holy Name. Whether one's knee is literally bowed or not, each time one reverently repeats the Holy Name of Jesus one can also offer Him a conscious act of worship, homage, honor, adoration, or reparation. For example, one can bow one's head slightly, or strike one's breast as the repentant publican did at the back of the temple (Lk 8:13). Similarly, if one is praying a decade of the rosary and counting off the ten prayers – one can count off each prayer upon uttering the name "Jesus".

In truth, on a daily basis, no one ever worshipped Jesus more than His own mother. And certainly she had a very special affection for her Son's name. If we today worship Jesus as we reverently repeat His name in prayer, we are simply imitating what His own mother did two thousand years ago. So Mary becomes the model for us as we focus on her Son, at the center of her life and at the heart of the "Hail Mary prayer". And indeed, in the last line of the prayer, when we are referring to the moment of our death, there is no doubt but that Jesus our Savior is the One whose mercy we seek, and we ask that the Savior's tender – dare we say persuasively tender – mother also seek that mercy on our behalf.

Such an approach can help the one who prays, as each prayer is built up, around the name, and Person, of Jesus, so that the focal point of the prayer is definitively "the fruit of thy womb, Jesus". The entire prayer emanates outward from the name of "Jesus" just as the spokes of a wheel extend outwards from the wheel's hub. Using this analogy, the other words of the prayer and our intentions together flow outwards as do the spokes of the wheel.

Finally, there is a certain power in the Name of Jesus (Acts 4:7-10) which empowers and drives this prayer from within. So that people praying to the mother of Jesus in this prayer are doing so based on their faith in Jesus and uniting themselves to Him and the power of His Name. So, whether the focus is on Unborn Jesus, Newborn Jesus or our Savior Jesus, He is Jesus the fruit of Mary's womb, and like Mary, we should have Him at the center of our lives.